INTRODUCTION TO DRUG ANALYSIS

Robert F. Raffauf, PhD
Professor of Medicinal Chemistry
Department of Medicinal Chemistry and Pharmacology
College of Pharmacy and Allied Health Professions
Northeastern University, Boston, Massachusetts

and

Victor D. Warner, PhD
Chairman, Department of Medicinal Chemistry and Pharmacology
College of Pharmacy and Allied Health Professions
Northeastern University, Boston, Massachusetts

F. A. DAVIS COMPANY, PHILADELPHIA

Printed in the United States of America

Library of Congress Cataloging in Publication Data

Raffauf, Robert Francis, 1916–
Introduction to drug analysis.

1. Drugs—Analysis. 2. Chemistry, Analytic.
I. Warner, Victor D., joint author. II. Title.
RS189.R33 615′.1901 77-11895
ISBN 0-8036-7250-0

Dedication

To those of our students whose suggestions and constructive criticism have been a great help in bringing this book to its present form.

Preface

In an environment which tends to emphasize the community and hospital aspects of pharmacy and the pharmacist's many opportunities to serve the customer or patient, students as well as faculty are inclined to question the relevance of analytical chemistry, drug analysis, or pharmaceutical analysis to the pharmacy curriculum. How much or how little of the theory of analytical chemistry, as well as "hands-on" laboratory experience, is necessary or desirable for today's student might be debated at some length.

In our view, justification of the position of drug analysis in the curriculum rests on three premises. First, all steps in the discovery, development, and use of drugs involve analytical principles. The pharmacist, as an expert educated in drugs and their uses, certainly should be familiar with and be able to talk intelligently about these principles and their application to pharmaceutical problems. Second, increased emphasis on clinical pharmacy and biopharmaceutics requires an understanding of the methods used, for example, in the determination of drug blood levels, and the limitations of these methods. Third, and we believe most important for the student, regardless of his career objectives, the thought processes involved in understanding equilibrium; pH and its control in biological systems; the solubility, absorption, and distribution of drugs; and oxidation-reduction as metabolic processes are all relevant to concepts to which he becomes exposed in other courses.

In answer to the question of whether or not a traditional course in analytical chemistry need be prerequisite to pharmaceutical analysis, we have taken the position that compounds are drugs only by reason of their ability to effect biological systems and that pharmaceutical analysis is analytical chemistry applied to a wide range of both inorganic and organic substances. Therefore, it seemed reasonable that the basic principles taught in modern courses in inorganic and organic chemistry as well as some material covered in the first courses in pharmacy itself would form a sufficiently strong base for a single course in analytical chemistry with emphasis on application to drug substances.

Almost without exception, students beginning their professional careers in pharmacy find analytical chemistry a difficult subject. There are several reasons for this. A large amount of material is covered in a comparatively short time. Course content is not of the type easily committed to memory for repetition on examinations. Analysis of any problem requires the accumulation of data, their interpretation, and their eventual use in making important decisions, a task often difficult for student and nonstudent alike. In spite of basic requirements and prerequisites, students come to their professional courses with a diversity of backgrounds. Some will have had strong, fundamental courses in freshman and organic chemistry, others will not. Some will retain some semblance of familiarity with basic mathematics; others will have forgotten logarithms and their uses as quickly as they were once learned.

For these reasons we have tried to construct a single course in which each concept is reduced to its simplest terms and emphasis is placed on the pharmaceutical applications of these concepts, at the same time providing the student with the background necessary for more advanced courses if he should choose them. Available textbooks have not proven entirely satisfactory for such an endeavor. We have written our text in lecture note style; class time is used to explore the thinking process, to learn to solve analytical problems, and to elaborate on the pharmaceutical applications of the analytical techniques covered in the course. This, we feel, places emphasis in the classroom, on the group situation, and on that material with which students have the most difficulty—the "how" of approaching problems.

Laboratory experiments are designed to give practical experience with the methods used in the United States Pharmacopeia, the National Formulary, or quality control applications. To avoid problems in the use of spectrometers, particularly with large laboratory sections, we have found it convenient to present the use of infrared, nuclear magnetic resonance, and mass spectrometers as demonstrations, and then to give our students prerecorded spectra of an "unknown" sample for interpretation in terms of a list of possible compounds which they are asked to identify. Instructors may wish to modify these experiments to suit their individual needs.

Although written primarily with the current needs of the pharmacy student in mind, it is hoped that this book will serve the student in related health sciences if not also the major in chemistry who would normally elect more advanced courses later in his academic career. The inclusion of more material than can be covered in a single course is intended to permit the individual instructor a latitude in emphasis which may be dictated by the content of other courses in the curriculum.

Robert F. Raffauf

Victor D. Warner

Contents

Laboratory Experiments

Chapter 1

Introduction

We might generalize about chemical analysis by saying that it deals with two questions: *what* a preparation contains *(qualitative analysis)* and *how much* of a given ingredient is present in a mixture, preparation, or sample *(quantitative analysis)*. In some cases, our ability to answer the first question may be limited by the quantity present; very special techniques may be required to identify a very small amount of an impurity in a sample or a very small amount of an active material in a tablet or capsule containing a relatively large amount of inert ingredients. Likewise, special methods may be necessary to measure the amounts of these things accurately should the need arise. In this course we will concentrate on the quantitative analysis of standard pharmaceutical preparations and the assay techniques used in the official drug compendia. We will also explore a few of the newer analytical techniques which have found places in hospital and clinical laboratories and which are becoming accepted methods in pharmaceutical analysis in its broadest sense.

The *methods* of analysis can be divided into rather simple categories for convenience:

1. Chemical methods, as the name implies, rely on the chemical reactions of atoms, ions, and molecules which proceed to quantitative conclusions and can therefore be used to determine the amount of substance present. These methods may be (a) gravimetric, in which the substance sought, or a derivative of it, may be separated from a mixture, dried, and weighed to determine the quantity present, or (b) volumetric, in which the amounts present can be determined by accurate measurement of volumes of reacting substances.

2. Physical methods are often used to establish criteria of purity of single substances; specific gravity, density, optical rotation, and refractive index are examples of these. Spectroscopic methods have increasing usefulness in the identification of drug substances as well as in the quantitative estimation of pharmaceutical preparations, body fluids, and the like.

Many analytical procedures are, of course, a combination of methods which depend to a greater or lesser degree on both the chemical and physical properties of drug molecules for their separation, detection, and estimation. As examples, we might mention the distribution of substances between immiscible solvents or the chromatographic separation of compounds from mixtures, either for their detection or their quantitative determination. This list is not complete but it covers the most important analytical tools with which the pharmacist will be concerned. The application of these methods will constitute the laboratory portion of this introductory course.

The *equipment* used in analytical chemistry is often specialized and somewhat different from the common glassware and instruments you may have used in previous courses. Many comprehensive analytical texts describe such equipment, and suppliers' catalogs and trade papers are often available in your chemistry library. You will have an opportunity to familiarize yourself with much of this equipment during the laboratory portion of the course. Whenever you are not sure of the proper use or care of a particular piece of apparatus, consult your laboratory instructor.

The *language* of analytical chemistry is essentially the language of chemistry itself, and it may be well to review briefly some of the terms, symbols, and concepts with which we will deal in our subsequent discussions. You will remember that matter is composed of *atoms* each of which is designated by an appropriate symbol. These atoms differ in weight, the *atomic weight,* which is assigned in relation to that of carbon, 12.000. You recall that atoms combine in definite proportions to form *molecules* which can react with other molecules and the weights of which *(molecular or formula weights)* are represented by the sum of the weights of the atoms of which they are composed. Usually the reactions we will study are carried out in solution so that we can speak correctly of the interaction of the *ions* involved expressed in the form of an *equation,* for example:

$$Ag^+ + Cl^- \rightarrow AgCl$$

These ions will react in the proportion described by their atomic weights and their *valence* or electrical charge so that one atomic weight of silver (107.8) will react with one atomic weight of chlorine (35.5) to yield one formula weight of silver chloride (143.3). We have chosen to describe this reaction in terms of the ions involved; actually, the silver may have come from silver nitrate and the chloride ion from sodium chloride so that a complete description of the process might look like this:

$$AgNO_3 \rightarrow Ag^+ + NO_3^-$$

$$NaCl \rightarrow Na^+ + Cl^-$$

Eq. 1 $$AgNO_3 + NaCl \rightarrow Na^+ + NO_3^- + AgCl \text{ (precipitate)}$$

To convert the relative weights to absolute weights, the chemist has coined the term *mole,* the atomic or molecular weight in grams. Thus, a mole of silver nitrate (169.8 gm.) reacts with 1 mole of sodium chloride (58.5 gm.) to form 1 mole of silver chloride (143.3 gm.), an insoluble precipitate which might be filtered from the solution and weighed in order to prove this, and 1 mole of sodium nitrate (85.0 gm.) as Na^+ and NO_3^-.

We have described this reaction by writing an *equation;* notice that the same number of atoms of each substance appears on either side of it. Now consider the reactions of silver nitrate with some other salts:

Eq. 2 $$2\,AgNO_3 + Na_2S \rightarrow Ag_2S + 2\,NaNO_3$$

Eq. 3 $$3\,AgNO_3 + Na_3PO_4 \rightarrow Ag_3PO_4 + 3\,NaNO_3$$

If we concentrate on the ions of particular interest, we may write:

$$2\,Ag^+ + S^= \rightarrow Ag_2S$$

$$3\,Ag^+ + PO_4^\equiv \rightarrow Ag_3PO_4$$

We see that 2 moles of silver nitrate are required to produce 1 mole of silver sulfide and that 3 moles are necessary to yield 1 mole of silver phosphate. With these concepts in mind, it is now possible to deal with some simple problems.

Example 1. How many grams of calcium chloride will react with 7.0 gm. of sodium sulfate to form calcium sulfate?

Solution. (a) Write and balance the equation for the reaction.

$$CaCl_2 + Na_2SO_4 \rightarrow CaSO_4 + 2\,NaCl$$

(b) Set up the proportion between the weights given and the formula weights.

$$\frac{x \text{ gm.}}{\text{f.w. } CaCl_2} = \frac{7.0 \text{ gm.}}{\text{f.w. } Na_2SO_4}$$

(c) Calculate the formula weights from the atomic weights and solve the equation.

$$\frac{x}{111} = \frac{7.0}{142}; \quad x = \frac{7.0 \times 111}{142} = 5.47 \text{ gm.}$$

Example 2. How many grams of silver would be required to give 4.18 gm. of silver phosphate?

Solution. This problem can be divided into two parts. First, the metallic silver must be dissolved, for example, using nitric acid:

$$2\,Ag^{\circ} + 2\,HNO_3 \rightarrow 2\,Ag^{+} + NO_3^{-} + H_2O + NO_2$$

The phosphate ion might be obtained from sodium phosphate.

$$Na_3PO_4 \rightarrow 3\,Na^{+} + PO_4^{\equiv}$$

Using only the ions of interest to express the final reaction,

$$3\,Ag^{+} + PO_4^{\equiv} \rightarrow Ag_3PO_4.$$

Then

$$\frac{x}{3(107.87)} = \frac{4.18}{418.4}$$

and

$$x = \frac{323.6 \times 4.18}{418.4} = 3.23 \text{ gm.}$$

The amounts of reacting substances which we have been considering, e.g., 1 mole (418 gm.) of silver phosphate, are inordinately large compared to those actually used in the usual analytical determinations. It is much more convenient to deal with 1/1000 of this amount, a *millimole*. This is simply the atomic or the formula weight in milligrams rather than grams.

We have said that most of our reactions will be carried out in solution, usually water, so that we must now introduce the concept of *concentration* to describe solutions which contain a specified amount of solute per given volume. There are several ways to express this. In the strict sense, we cannot prepare a solution containing 1 mole of NaCl or $AgNO_3$; these are nearly completely ionized salts which exist in solution as Na^+, Cl^-, Ag^+, and NO_3^- ions and the concentration of NaCl and $AgNO_3$ as such is very low. Strictly speaking, the concentrations of these solutions should be expressed in terms of *formality* (F) representing the number of gram-formula weights per liter of solution. The term *molarity* (M) is used to express the actual concentration of the ions and/or the undissociated species in a particular solution and thus represents the equilibrium concentration. We will be dealing primarily with equilibria and will use the latter term, keeping in mind the distinction between the two. Thus, in Eq. 1 it is clear that a solution 1 M in Ag^+ will react completely with a solution 1 M in Cl^-, but that in Eqs. 2 and 3, two and three times the volume of 1 M Ag^+ would be required for the complete reaction with 1 M sulfide and phosphate respectively.

Another way to state this is to say that 1 mole of Ag^+ will react with 0.5 mole of $S^=$ or 0.33 mole of $PO_4^{\equiv}$. The *equivalent weights* of Na_2S and Na_3PO_4 used in these reactions with $AgNO_3$ would be $Na_2S/2$ and $Na_3PO_4/3$. Solutions containing an equivalent weight per liter, or a milliequivalent per milliliter, are called *normal* (N) solutions. When using this method of expressing concentration, a degree of caution is required for in simple displacement reactions normality depends on the number of replaceable hydrogen or hydroxyl ions (acid-base titrations) or on the valence of the specific ion in question (precipitation reactions). We will discuss the special case of oxidation-reduction reactions in due course.

A few examples will make these distinctions clear. If we were to titrate but one of the two replaceable H^+ ions in sulfuric acid (H_2SO_4) according to

$$H_2SO_4 + NaOH \rightarrow NaHSO_4 + H_2O,$$

its equivalent weight would be its formula weight; whereas if both H^+ were titrated according to

$$H_2SO_4 + NaOH \rightarrow Na_2SO_4 + 2\ H_2O,$$

its equivalent weight would be $H_2SO_4/2$ and a solution containing 49 gm./L. would be 0.5 M or 1.0 N.

In the complete precipitation of aluminum as its hydroxide by ammonia, the following equation holds:

$$AlCl_3 + 3\ NH_4OH \rightarrow Al(OH)_3 + 3\ NH_4Cl$$

Can you see that a given volume of a 1.0 M solution of aluminum chloride would require three volumes of ammonia solution of the same molarity and that equal volumes of a 1.0 N solution of each reagent would complete the precipitation as described?

Example 3. How many grams of Na_3PO_4 would be required to prepare a liter of 0.1 N solution to be used in a reaction according to Eq. 3 (p. 2)?

Solution. 1 equivalent = $Na_3PO_4/3 = 163.94/3 = 54.65$ gm.
A 0.1 N solution contains $0.1 \times 54.7 = 5.47$ gm./L.

Example 4. Had a liter of 0.1 M solution been required, the amount of Na_3PO_4 to be used would be simply $0.1 \times 163.9 = 16.4$ gm.

Some of the typical problems encountered in practice are more complex and depend on a sound knowledge of these relationships for their solution.

Example 5. Sodium Chloride Injection (U.S.P. XIX, 456) contains 0.9 percent w/v NaCl. Calculate the molarity of such a solution.

Solution. We will assume that 100 ml. of water weighs 100 gm. Then a 0.9 percent solution of sodium chloride contains 0.9 gm./100 ml. or 9.0 gm./L. By the definitions we have given, a 0.1 M solution contains 22.99 (Na) + 35.45 (Cl) = 58.44 gm./L. Our solution contains 9.0 gm./L.; its molarity is therefore 9.0/58.44 = 0.154 M.

Example 6. Barium sulfate is a radiopaque medium used in radiography of the gastrointestinal tract. It can be prepared by precipitation from a solution of barium chloride using sulfuric acid. A solution of $BaCl_2$ was treated with 40.00 ml. of dilute solution of H_2SO_4 to give 1.2345 gm. of $BaSO_4$. Calculate for the sulfuric acid solution (a) grams of H_2SO_4 per liter and (b) the molarity.

Solution. The equation representing this reaction is:

$$BaCl_2 + H_2SO_4 \rightarrow 2\,HCl + BaSO_4\downarrow$$

This tells us that for every mole of $BaSO_4$ produced, we will need an equal number of moles of H_2SO_4 to produce it. We obtained 1.2345 gm. of the product, 1 mole of which would weigh 137.34 (Ba) + 32.06 (S) + 64.00 (O_4) = 233.4 gm. We obtained, then, 1.2345/233.4 = 0.0053 mole which would require 0.0053 × 98.06 = 0.5197 gm. H_2SO_4. This was contained in 40.00 ml. of solution representing (1000 × 0.5197)/40.00 = 12.99 gm./L. or (1000 × 0.0053)/40.00 = 0.133 moles/L. or 0.133 M.

Example 7. The object of a particular experiment was to determine the percent purity of a sample of oxalic acid dihydrate the formula for which is $C_2H_2O_4 \cdot 2\,H_2O$. The laboratory notebook contained the following data:

Weight of sample + weighing paper	0.7770 gm.
Weight of weighing paper	0.3020 gm.
Weight of sample	0.4750 gm.
Milliliters of 0.2000 N NaOH used	35.60

Solution. This problem can be solved in two ways. Oxalic acid is a dibasic acid (HOOC-COOH) and has two replaceable H^+ ions. Its neutralization is expressed by the following equation:

$$H_2C_2O_4 + 2\,NaOH \rightarrow Na_2C_2O_4 + 2\,H_2O$$

Two moles of sodium hydroxide are required per mole of oxalic acid. It is easier to use millimoles. For sodium hydroxide, which has one replaceable OH^- ion, molarity equals normality; therefore 35.60 ml. × 0.2000 M = 7.12 mM. used. But according to the equation each millimole corresponds to 0.5 mM. of oxalic acid; 7.12 mM. NaOH = 3.56 mM. oxalic acid. One millimole of oxalic acid dihydrate (don't forget the water of crystallization!) = 126.08; 3.56 × 126.08 = 448.8 mg. = 0.4488 gm. The sample was 0.4750 gm. It was therefore (0.4488/0.4750) × 100 = 94.5 percent pure. Using milliequivalents leads, of course, to the same result:

$$35.60 \times 0.2000 = 7.12 \text{ mEq. NaOH}$$

which is equal to the milliequivalents of oxalic acid titrated, and because it has two replaceable H^+ ions, 1 mEq. of oxalic acid = 63.04 mg.; 7.12 mEq. = 7.12 × 63.04 = 448.8 mg. Calculation of percent purity is done in the same manner as above.

THINGS TO REMEMBER

MOLE = molecular (formula) weight in grams
MILLIMOLE = molecular weight in milligrams
MOLAR = solution containing a mole per liter
EQUIVALENT WEIGHT = formula weight ÷ valence of reacting ion(s)
NORMAL = solution containing an equivalent weight per liter
MOLES = liters × molarity (M)
MILLIMOLES (mM.) = milliliters × molarity
EQUIVALENTS (Eq.) = liters × normality (N)
MILLIEQUIVALENTS (mEq.) = milliliters × normality
Two solutions of different normality relate to each other as follows:

$$\text{ml.}_1 \times N_1 = \text{ml.}_2 \times N_2$$

PROBLEMS

1. How many grams of hydrogen would be obtained by reacting completely 5.0 gm. of zinc with hydrochloric acid?
2. How many milliliters of (a) 2.00 M HCl and (b) 2.00 N HCl would be necessary to dissolve 5.00 gm. of zinc?
3. What is the maximum weight of sodium chloride which could be obtained from 10.000 gm. of pure sodium hydroxide?
4. A sulfuric acid solution contained 50.11 gm. H_2SO_4/L. Of this, 42.27 ml. required 45.28 ml. of KOH to neutralize it. Calculate the normality of the KOH solution.
5. Boric Acid Vehicle (U.S.P. XIX, 703) is prepared by dissolving 1.90 gm. of H_3BO_3 in sufficient water to make 100 ml. of solution. Calculate the molarity and the normality of this vehicle.
6. A solution of a base is known to be exactly 0.1175 N. How much water should be added to 1 L. in order to make it exactly 0.0950 N?
7. A piece of impure silver wire weighing 0.1000 gm. was dissolved in nitric acid thus converting it to silver nitrate. After dilution with water, the solution was treated with a dilute solution of sodium chloride until all of the Ag^+ had been precipitated as AgCl (0.1010 gm.). Calculate the percent purity of the silver.

8. A sample of powder containing some sodium carbonate (Na_2CO_3) weighed 5.00 gm. It was treated with an excess of sulfuric acid, and the liberated carbon dioxide was bubbled into a solution of barium hydroxide ($Ba(OH)_2$) to form 0.4600 gm. of $BaCO_3$. Calculate the percentage of sodium carbonate in the powder.
9. A bottle that had a label that was no longer completely legible was known to contain either chlorobenzene (C_6H_5Cl) or benzyl chloride (C_7H_7Cl). A sample weighing 0.1500 gm. was decomposed to convert all chlorine to chloride which was then precipitated with $AgNO_3$ to yield 0.1906 gm. of AgCl. What is the percentage of chlorine in the sample? Which of the two possibilities is it?
10. One of the forms of Dextrose Injection (U.S.P. XIX, 129) is a 10 percent solution of glucose monohydrate, $C_6H_{12}O_6 \cdot H_2O$. You have a bottle of sterile 2.5 M glucose monohydrate solution. How would you prepare a liter of the U.S.P. solution?
11. A 5.00 gm. sample of a monobasic acid was dissolved in water to make 100 ml. of solution. A 25.00 ml. portion was titrated with 0.200 N NaOH, 51.00 ml. being used. Calculate the molecular weight of the acid.

ANSWERS

1. 0.15 gm.
2. 76.5 ml.
3. 14.625 gm.
4. 0.954 N
5. 0.308 M; 0.924 N
6. 236.8 ml.
7. 76.0 percent
8. 4.94 percent
9. 31.43 percent; chlorobenzene
10. dilute 202 ml. of 2.5 M to 1 L.
11. 123

Chapter 2

Some Simple Mathematics

LOGARITHMS AND THEIR USES

The availability of the pocket calculator certainly has simplified the performance of routine calculations necessary in analytical chemistry. Nonetheless, it is appropriate to review a few of the basic operations involving exponential notation which is commonly used for many of the very small or very large numbers used in these calculations. You will recall that numbers can be expressed as powers of 10:

$$1000 = 10^3$$
$$100 = 10^2$$
$$1 = 10^0$$
$$0.01 = 10^{-2}$$
$$0.0001 = 10^{-4}$$

The exponent, the power to which 10 must be raised to give the number, is called the logarithm: if $n = 10^x$ then $\log n = x$. Remember, too, that multiplication or division of numbers expressed this way is simply a matter of adding or subtracting the exponents, so that

$$10^2 \times 10^3 = 10^5 = 100000$$
$$10^{-2} \times 10^{-3} = 10^{-5} = 0.00001$$
$$10^{-2} \times 10^3 = 10^1 = 10$$

or $\dfrac{10^5}{10^2} = 10^3 = 1000$, and $\dfrac{10^{-5}}{10^2} = 10^{-7} = 0.0000001$. Numbers raised to a given power are easily calculated by multiplying exponents:

$$100^3 = (10^2)^3 = 10^6 = 1{,}000{,}000$$
$$(0.01)^3 = (10^{-2})^3 = 10^{-6} = 0.000001$$

Roots are obtained by dividing exponents:

$$\sqrt{10^6} = 10^3 = 1000$$
$$\sqrt[3]{10^{-6}} = 10^{-2} = 0.01$$
$$\sqrt[4]{10^{12}} = 10^3 = 1000$$

Whole powers of 10 are handled simply enough. Do you remember how to deal with numbers that are not whole powers of 10? It is clear that a number such as 550 lies somewhere between 100 (10^2) and 1000 (10^3); its exponent is fractional. Look at it in this way:

$$550 = 5.5 \times 100 = 5.5 \times 10^2$$

Since the logarithm of a product is the sum of the logarithms of the numbers multiplied, we can say:

$$\begin{aligned}\log 550 &= \log 5.5 + \log 10^2\\ &= 0.740 + 2\\ &= 2.740\end{aligned}$$

or $550 = 10^{2.740}$. The logarithm (2.740) is composed of two parts, the characteristic (2) and the mantissa (0.740), and may be found in tables published in many texts and handbooks.

Then, given a number, what is its logarithm? Consider, for example, 0.00027. This can be expressed as 2.7×10^{-4}, and

$$\begin{aligned}\log 2.7 \times 10^{-4} &= \log 2.7 + \log 10^{-4}\\ &= 0.432 + (-4)\\ & -3.368\end{aligned}$$

A solution to the reverse problem is often required: given a logarithm, to what number does it correspond?

$$\begin{aligned}\log n &= 2.740\\ n &= 10^2 \times 10^{0.740}\end{aligned}$$

The number corresponding to $10^2 = 100$; that corresponding to $10^{0.740} = 5.5$; $n = 100 \times 5.5 = 550$. Now, what if $\log n = -3.568$? We cannot look up negative logarithms in the tables, but we can break them into two powers of 10 as follows:

$$\begin{aligned}n &= 10^{-4} \times 10^{0.432}\\ &= 10^{-4} \times 2.70\\ &= 0.0001 \times 2.70\\ &= 0.00027\end{aligned}$$

To see how this might work in a practical situation, we can solve the problem of the titration of oxalic acid (Example 7, p. 5) using moles and liters instead of millimoles and milliliters.

$$35.60 \text{ ml.} = 0.0356 \text{ L.}$$

$$\text{Moles} = \text{L.} \times \text{M} = 0.0356 \times 0.2000$$

or $(3.56 \times 10^{-2})(2 \times 10^{-1}) = 7.12 \times 10^{-3}$ moles of NaOH used which is equivalent to 3.56×10^{-3} moles of oxalic acid titrated. One mole of oxalic acid dihydrate = 126.08 gm.; total amount of oxalic acid is therefore $(1.2608 \times 10^{2})(3.56 \times 10^{-3}) = 4.488 \times 10^{-1} = 0.4488$ gm. Such calculations are common in analytical chemistry; familiarity with them can be gained through practice with the problems at the end of this chapter.

ERRORS AND TREATMENT OF ANALYTICAL DATA

Surely we all agree that among the goals of truly professional practice are that the manufacturer produce and the pharmacist dispense quality products of known purity, in carefully regulated doses, and in some reproducible form on which the physician, and especially the patient, can depend. The United States Pharmacopeia and National Formulary exist to insure such standards and to their maintenance the analyst brings a constant concern. Yet, we must admit that a *completely* truthful statement of the composition of a particular preparation is difficult, if not impossible. This is so because of the intrusion of various *errors* into the long chain of events beginning with the manufacturing process and ending, possibly, with the labelling of the prescription. We shall concern ourselves primarily with those arising in the analytical procedure.

Errors are of two types: *Systematic* or *determinate* errors are those which may be due to an inadequate method, faulty equipment, uncalibrated glassware, impure or off-standard reagents, or errors on the part of the operator. They may be reduced or eliminated by careful attention to these details. There remain, however, *random* or *indeterminate* errors which are sometimes called accidental errors in the sense that they are not predictable but exist because there is a degree of uncertainty in all measurements and observations. Such errors cannot be eliminated, but they can be minimized by statistical methods.

We need not deal here with the intricacies of the mathematics of probability and statistical calculations except to learn a few of the basic concepts and terms applicable to the work of this course.

Accuracy is the degree to which the determined result agrees with the true value. In a very real sense, we are never really certain of the true value; the analyst's job is to come as close to it as possible so that, with a high degree of probability, he can express something close to the true value. In other words, we can look upon accuracy as a reflection of the agreement between a measured value and an accepted true value for that which is measured. *Precision,* on the other hand, is a measure of the degree to which a determination can be repeated in successive experiments, whether the result is accurate or not. It is a measure of reproducibility.

To discover and understand the relationships between these concepts and their bearing on the analytical result, it is necessary to recognize that the result of an analysis is usually a set of figures—multiple determinations of the number of grams in a given volume of solution, percent purity of a sample, or even grade point averages!

Significant figures are defined as the digits necessary to express the result of a measurement to the precision with which it was made. This precision depends on the purpose the measurement is intended to serve. You would be unlikely to use a bathroom scale capable of giving your body weight to the nearest ounce or to count out prescribed tablets to the nearest half-dozen. In the first instance, the degree of precision would be much higher than necessary, while in the second it would certainly not be high enough. An idea of what we mean by significant figures can be gained from the examples in columns I and II below:

I	II
1.25 gm.	1.2466 gm.
125 lbs.	124.66 lbs.
1.25 L.	1.2466 L.

It is clear that the measurements in column II (five significant figures) were made with instruments having a greater sensitivity than were those in column I (three significant figures). Very large or very small numbers require special notice. Consider 1,000,000 and 0.000001. These can be expressed exponentially as 1×10^6 and 1×10^{-6}, respectively. There is only one significant figure in each term. Zeros used to fix the decimal point are *not* significant figures. There is one significant figure in 0.01, there are three in 0.0102, four in 1.004 and two in 0.0020. In the last case, the final zero is significant because it indicates that the result was neither 0.0019 nor 0.0021, but it might have been 0.00199 or 0.00201. To this extent, the last digit in a figure is uncertain. You will see this expressed, for example, as 11.5 ± 0.1 gm. This we call *absolute uncertainty;* it is expressed directly in the units of measurement, and the expression simply states that the value was equal to or greater than 11.4 but equal to or less than 11.6 gm. As another example we might take a buret reading of 25.0 ml. This tells us that the reading was between 24.9 and 25.1 ml., and we may write the value as 25.0 ± 0.1 ml. However, the *relative uncertainty* in these measurements is quite different. This is expressed in terms of the magnitude of the measurement and would be one part in 115 in the first case, and one part in 250 in the second. Notice that if we were to read the buret to the nearest 0.05 ml., and this is possible for most operators, we might have recorded the volume as 25.05 ml. (25.05 ± 0.05) and, though the last digit is uncertain, the relative uncertainty of the measurement is now one part in 501. You may see relative uncertainty expressed in parts per hundred (percent), parts per thousand (p.p.t.), or parts per million (p.p.m.).

Consider a few more examples of the use of these concepts. The following is a typical entry in a laboratory notebook:

Weight of sample + paper	0.7124 gm.
Weight of paper	0.2123 gm.
Weight of sample	0.5001 gm.

There are four significant figures in all of these data, an indication of the sensitivity of the balance used for the weighings. The absolute uncertainty is 0.0001 gm. in all cases, but the relative uncertainties are 1/7124, 1/2123, and 1/5001, respectively, for these measurements. We can summarize the importance of these concepts to analytical calculations in a few simple rules:

1. The result of a series of mathematical operations on a group of numbers cannot be stated more precisely than the least precise number in the group.

2. When adding or subtracting quantities, they should be measured to the same absolute uncertainty.

3. When multiplying or dividing quantities, they should be measured to the same relative uncertainty.

Another example involves the calculation of the formula weight for sodium bicarbonate ($NaHCO_3$) from an atomic weight table:

$$\begin{aligned} \text{Na} &= 22.9898 \\ \text{H} &= 1.00797 \\ \text{C} &= 12.01115 \\ 3 \times \text{O} &= \underline{47.9982} \\ & 84.00712 \end{aligned}$$

The limiting terms are the atomic weights of Na and O which are not known with the same certainty as the others. The answer is therefore 84.0071.

Looking at this mathematical operation

$$\frac{37.25 \times 0.5270}{1.2345} = 15.901782$$

we can see that the relative uncertainty is determined by the term 37.25 (one part in 3725). Since the answer cannot be more certain than this, 15.90 is the correct expression of the answer.

With these details in mind, how can we approach more closely a true or accepted value for an analytical determination? Since indeterminate errors are random, we can do multiple determinations and, relying on the fact that at least in part these random errors tend to cancel each other out, we can treat the result by a few simple statistical methods. Suppose, in titrating an acid with standard sodium hydroxide, the following data were obtained:

$$\begin{aligned} \text{NaOH used (ml.)} &= 22.60\ (X_1) \\ & 22.55\ (X_2) \\ & 22.70\ (X_3) \\ & 22.20\ (X_4) \end{aligned}$$

$$\text{mean or average} = (\overline{X}) = 90.05 \div 4 = 22.51 \text{ ml.}$$

We can now make an assessment of the precision of our observations. One way to do this is to compute the *average deviation* $(\overline{d})$. This is done as follows:

$$\begin{aligned} X_1 - \overline{X} &= 22.60 - 22.51 = +0.09 = d_1 \\ X_2 - \overline{X} &= 22.55 - 22.51 = +0.04 = d_2 \\ X_3 - \overline{X} &= 22.70 - 22.51 = +0.19 = d_3 \\ X_4 - \overline{X} &= 22.20 - 22.51 = -0.31 = d_4 \end{aligned}$$

Neglecting the algebraic signs, the average of these deviations $(\overline{d})$ is 0.16. A better measure of the precision is the *standard deviation (s)* which is defined as the square root of the sum of the squares of the individual deviations divided by the number of measurements. In practice, if the number of measurements is less than 10, better results can be obtained by dividing by one less than the number of measurements. Using the example above,

d	d^2
0.09	0.0081
0.04	0.0016
0.19	0.0361
0.31	0.0961
	0.1419

Now, $s = \sqrt{\Sigma d^2/n - 1} = \sqrt{0.1419/3} = \sqrt{0.0473} = 0.2175 = 0.22.$

The significance of s is that, by appropriate mathematics, it can be shown that 95 percent of all values may be expected to fall within the limits of $\pm 2s$. This is strictly true only after an infinite number of observations. In the example we have used, we might expect 95 percent of all titrations to use 22.51 ± 0.44 ml. of NaOH, provided, of course, that no determinate errors occurred during the course of the analysis.

At first glance, the preceding results seem to indicate a "poor" experiment; the observation X_4 appears "out of line" and is certainly lower than the others. For the method, and with a competent operator, we should be able to expect better precision. How close do results have to agree (precision) in order that we accept them as an estimate of the true result (accuracy)? Or to put it another way, on what basis can we reject a suspected "poor" result?

We have just seen that we might reject a result that does not fall within $\pm 2s$. On this basis, the suspected low value of 22.20 ml. might be acceptable. There is another way to arrive at this decision. If it is not possible to run another analysis, perhaps due to lack of sample, and having checked the method and his interpretation of it and the experimental directions, the analyst might then run a so-called "Q test." This is done as follows.

1. Arrange the results in decreasing order of value.
2. Record the range, i.e., the highest minus the lowest value.
3. Divide the difference between the suspected value and its nearest neighbor by the range.
4. Using this ratio (Q), consult an appropriate table for the confidence with which the suspected result may be accepted or rejected.

Such tables for many degrees of confidence may be found in many texts and handbooks. Table 1 is a brief listing of rejection quotients (Q values) at 90 percent confidence limits which will be sufficient for our purposes. If the Q value determined by steps 1 through 4 above is *larger* than the value given in Table 1 for the number of observations, the suspect observation may be rejected. Go through these calculations for the example we have cited; you will find that Q = 0.70 indicating that the apparent low value may be kept in calculation of the true result.

An example of a practical problem to which such data might be applied is the following:

Example. The results from an analysis of a 1:20,000 solution of Zephiran gave these values: 0.004986, 0.004989, 0.004992, and 0.004972 percent. Calculate: (a) the average deviation, (b) the standard deviation, (c) the absolute uncertainty of the average percent concentration, (d) the relative uncertainty of the average percent concentration, and (e) using the Q test, decide if the last value in the series should be rejected.

Solution. First calculate the average value for the series of results; you should find this to be, $\bar{X} = 0.004985$. Now subtract this average from each of the individual observations to obtain the deviations (d) and, neglecting the algebraic signs, average these to obtain (a) the

Table 1. Rejection Quotients with 90 percent Confidence Limits

Observations	*Q*
3	0.94
4	0.76
5	0.64
6	0.56
7	0.51
8	0.47

average deviation, $(\bar{d}) = 0.00000625 = 0.000006$ percent. To calculate the standard deviation it is more convenient to use exponential notation:

$$d_1^2 = (1 \times 10^{-6})^2 = 1 \times 10^{-12}$$

$$d_2^2 = (4 \times 10^{-6})^2 = 16 \times 10^{-12}$$

$$d_3^2 = (7 \times 10^{-6})^2 = 49 \times 10^{-12}$$

$$d_4^2 = (13 \times 10^{-6})^2 = 169 \times 10^{-12}$$

$$\Sigma d^2 = 235 \times 10^{-12} \quad \text{and} \quad s = \sqrt{235 \times 10^{-12}/3} = \sqrt{78.3 \times 10^{-12}} = 8.85 \times 10^{-6}$$

or (b), the standard deviation, is 0.000009 percent. Absolute uncertainty is given in the units measured. The average percent found under (a) was 0.004985; (c), the absolute uncertainty of the average percent concentration, must then be ±0.000001 percent; and (d), the relative uncertainty of the average percent concentration, is one part in 4985. For part (e) of the problem, the Q test, it is more convenient to omit the many zeros. Arrange the numbers in the highest to lowest order: 4992, 4989, 4986, 4972. The range is 20; the difference between the lowest (suspect) value and its nearest neighbor is 14; Q = 14/20 = 0.7. This value is below that given in the table for four observations so it can be kept in our calculations with 90 percent confidence that it is an acceptable value.

THINGS TO REMEMBER

If n = 10^x log n = x

ACCURACY: Agreement with true value

PRECISION: Reproducibility of result

SIGNIFICANT FIGURES: Digits necessary to express a result to the proper precision

AVERAGE DEVIATION: $\Sigma d/n$

STANDARD DEVIATION: $\sqrt{\Sigma d^2/n - 1}$

Experiment 1. The Analytical Balance

You will be given instruction in the use of the particular type of analytical balance which you will use throughout the laboratory portion of the course. Familiarize yourself with the balance and its controls. Ask your instructor to explain anything you do not understand concerning its use. Place a weighing bottle on the balance pan and determine its weight.

Using small forceps, transfer one of the tablets provided to the weighing bottle and record the new weight. Determine the weight of the tablet. Repeat this by weighing each of four additional tablets.

From the data you have obtained, calculate: (a) the average weight per tablet, (b) the average deviation in weight, (c) the standard deviation, (d) the range within which you can be 95 percent certain of the weight of any given tablet taken from the stock bottle. Record your results in the form prescribed by your instructor for this experiment.

PROBLEMS

1. Express the following numbers as powers of 10:
   (a) 1250, (b) 0.56, (c) 274, (d) 0.000015.
2. Convert these expressions to their corresponding numbers:
   (a) 3.5×10^6, (b) 1.8×10^{-5}, (c) $10^{-3.2}$, (d) $10^{4.5}$
3. Give the value for x in the following:
   (a) $x = (4 \times 10^{-4})^2$, (b) $x^2 = 25 \times 10^6$, (c) $3x^3 = 81 \times 10^{-9}$, (d) $x = \sqrt[4]{16 \times 10^4}$
4. Find the logarithms of the following numbers:
   (a) 0.01, (b) 1725, (c) 3.86, (d) 2001
5. The following logarithms represent numbers; find the numbers:
   (a) 3.650, (b) −2.12, (c) 0.950, (d) −0.836
6. How many significant figures are in each of the following numbers?
   (a) 0.0004, (b) 95.65, (c) 3.5×10^3
7. Calculate the molecular weight of boric acid (H_3BO_3) to the correct number of significant figures.
8. A student standardized a sample of KOH solution with the following results for its normality: 0.9987, 1.0002, 1.0000, 0.9998. Calculate the average deviation in parts per thousand and the standard deviation of the mean.
9. In a particular titration, the following buret readings were made: 25.05, 25.15, 25.35, 25.20. Which of these results, if any, should be rejected due to accidental error?
10. Four aspirin tablets were selected at random for assay. They weighed 0.3001, 0.3015, 0.3053, and 0.2985 gm. The mean value for the purity of the tablets after assay was 99.5 percent aspirin. Using the appropriate number of significant figures, calculate the number of milligrams of aspirin present in the average tablet. What is the average deviation in the weights of these tablets? What is the standard deviation?
11. How many milligrams of $Ca(OH)_2$ would be required to prepare 150 ml. of a 0.0250 N solution?
12. Express the results of the following calculations to the proper number of significant figures:
    (a) $1.060 + 0.05974 - 0.0013$
    (b) $2.5 \times 101{,}562.0$
    (c) $\dfrac{27.5 \times 13.0 \times 10.0}{(4.062 + 12.001)}$
    (d) $(3.456 \times 10^{-4})(2.4 \times 10^{-4})$

ANSWERS

1. (a) 1.250×10^3
   (b) 5.6×10^{-1}
   (c) 2.74×10^2
   (d) 1.5×10^{-5}
2. (a) 3500000
   (b) 0.000018
   (c) 0.000631
   (d) 31630
3. (a) 1.6×10^{-7}
   (b) 5×10^3
   (c) 3×10^{-3}
   (d) 2×10^1
4. (a) −2.000
   (b) 3.2367
   (c) 0.5866
   (d) 3.3012
5. (a) 4460
   (b) 0.0076
   (c) 8.90
   (d) 0.146
6. (a) one
   (b) four
   (c) two
7. 61.83
8. $\bar{d} = 0.5$ p.p.t.
   $s = 7 \times 10^{-4}$
9. None
10. 300 mg.
    $d = 2.1$ mg.
    $s = 0.0029$
11. 139 mg.
12. (a) 1.118
    (b) 250,000
    (c) 230
    (d) 8.3×10^{-8}

Chapter 3

Chemical Equilibrium—Acids and Bases

Certain chemical reactions with which you are familiar proceed to a definite conclusion. You may remember, for example, an experiment in freshman chemistry which involved the preparation of hydrogen by dissolving zinc in hydrochloric acid:

$$Zn^{\circ} + 2\,HCl \rightarrow H_2\uparrow + ZnCl_2$$

When all of the zinc had dissolved and the hydrogen had bubbled out of the solution, the reaction was finished. The same is true for reactions which form insoluble precipitates:

$$Ba^{++} + SO_4^{=} \rightarrow BaSO_4\downarrow$$

or those which form stable complexes:

$$2\,Ag^{+} + 2\,CN^{-} \rightarrow [Ag(CN)_2]^{-} + Ag^{+}.$$

In such reactions, the net result is the removal of one or both of the reactants from the solution so that no further chemical change can take place. Such reactions are essentially *irreversible*.

REVERSIBLE EQUILIBRIUM REACTIONS

In many other reactions such is not the case. These we can represent in a general way, $A + B \leftrightarrows C + D$, as reactions in which the products might recombine, in part, to reform the reactants. Such *reversible* reactions are said to reach equilibrium, a steady state in which both the forward and the reverse reactions are proceeding at a fixed rate. This state of affairs can be described by the *Law of Chemical Equilibrium:*

> In an equilibrium, the product of the total concentration of the resulting substances (products), divided by the product of the total concentration of the reactants—each concentration being raised to a power equal to the number of molecules entering into the reaction as shown by the equation for the reaction—is constant (K_{eq}) at constant temperature, pressure and concentration.

Thus, if $nA + mB \leftrightarrows xC + yD$, then

$$K_{eq} = \frac{[C]^x [D]^y}{[A]^n [B]^m}$$

The square brackets indicate molar concentration. We should note here that the theory of the nature of solutions of electrolytes in water dictates that, because of various interactions between the ions of the solute and the solvent, the real or effective concentration is somewhat different from the ideal concentration (molarity, normality) of which we usually speak. The expression which takes these effects into account is called the *activity (a)*. However, because in solutions of moderate concentration activity is proportional to concentration and because in dilute solutions the effects of ionic and molecular interaction are small enough to be negligible, we can use molar concentration for the analytical determinations with which we will be concerned.

Reversible equilibria form the basis of many analytical methods. One of the most important of these involves acids and bases. For most practical purposes we will be dealing with equilibrium reactions taking place in aqueous solutions. Under these conditions we can define an *acid* as a substance which can *donate* a proton and a *base* as a substance which can *accept* one. One cannot exist without the other:

Eq. 1 $$HCl + H_2O \leftrightarrows H_3O^+ + Cl^-$$

Eq. 2 $$NH_3 + H_2O \leftrightarrows NH_4^+ + OH^-$$

In Equation 1, HCl (an acid) donates its proton to water (a base) to form the hydronium ion (an acid) and the chloride ion (a base). In Equation 2, ammonia (a base) accepts a proton from water (an acid) to give the ammonium ion (an acid) and the hydroxide ion (a base). We speak of these as conjugate acid-base pairs. To become more familiar with the idea, go through the same reasoning for these reactions reading from right to left. Notice, however, that water plays a different role in each of the reactions. It can function either as an acid or a base, as a proton donor or acceptor, depending on circumstances. It is said to be *amphoteric*.

$$2\,H_2O \leftrightarrows H_3O^+ + OH^-$$

or simply $$H_2O \leftrightarrows H^+ + OH^-$$

This equilibrium, as opposed to that for HCl above, lies far to the left because water is but slightly ionized while HCl is completely so in dilute solution.

It should be clear that if we are to use such equilibria for quantitative analysis, we must have some method for determining the extent of this ionization or the concentration of ions in solution. It should be clear also that, since these are equilibria, we can apply the Law of Chemical Equilibrium to them as we did in a general way earlier. Thus, if $AB \leftrightarrows A^+ + B^-$, then $[A^+][B^-]/[AB] = K_{eq}$. In this case K_{eq} is called the *ionization constant* (K_i). Methods for the determination of these constants will be considered later in the course. For the moment we will be satisfied with a few examples of their application.

Consider the special case of water which, as we have seen, functions either as an acid or a base. Referring to the equation for the ionization of water above, we see that

$$\frac{[H^+]\,[OH^-]}{[H_2O]} = K_i$$

which you may see more commonly designated as K_w. The ionization constant for pure water has been determined to be 1×10^{-14}. In aqueous solutions $[H_2O]$ can be taken as unity, and since $[H^+] = [OH^-] = x$, it follows that

$$x^2 = K_w = 10^{-14}$$

$$\text{and} \qquad x = 10^{-7}$$

That is to say that 1 mole of water ionizes to give 10^{-7} mole of H^+ and 10^{-7} mole of OH^-.

The expression 0.0000001 M, or even 10^{-7}, can be cumbersome. A simpler method for referring to the hydrogen (or hydroxyl) concentration is desirable, especially because of its common use in analytical, biological, chemical, and pharmaceutical systems. The familiar expression *pH* is used for the purpose.

$$pH = \log 1/[H^+] = -\log [H^+]$$

Therefore, the pH of pure water is 7.00, this being by definition a *neutral* solution. Using the same notation, $pK_w = -\log K_w = 14.00$, and $pOH = pK_w - pH = 7.00$. This is just another way of expressing the neutrality of water—the equality of its acidic and basic character. Solutions which have a pH value higher than 7.00 are *alkaline;* those with lower values are *acidic*.

STRONG ACIDS AND BASES

Now let us examine a number of cases in which this concept might be applied. *Strong acids and bases* present no particular problem. These substances are completely ionized in dilute solution; at usual analytical concentrations all of the H^+ (or OH^-) in the solution will be due to their ionization, and the contribution to the total ion concentration due to the ionization of water will usually be so small as to be negligible.

Suppose we had a 0.0001 M solution of HCl. The concentration of H^+ due to the ionization of the acid is obviously $0.0001 = 10^{-4}$ M and the pH = 4.00. The pOH, were we interested in this, would be $14.00 - 4.00 = 10.00$.

Example 1. What is the pH of a 0.002 M solution of HCl?

Solution $[H^+] = 2 \times 10^{-3}$; $pH = -\log [H^+] = -\log 2 + (-\log 10^{-3})$

$$\text{or} \qquad pH = -\log 2 + 3 = -0.30 + 3.00$$

$$= 2.70$$

Another example, somewhat more complicated, can be given as follows:

Example 2. If 2 gm. of sodium hydroxide are dissolved in water to make 1 L. of solution, what is the pH?

Solution. 2 gm. NaOH = 2.0/40.0 mole = 0.05 mole/L. or 5×10^{-2} M. In such a solution $[OH^-] = 5 \times 10^{-2}$ and pOH would be $-\log 5 + 2.0 = 1.30$ and $pH = 14.00 - 1.30 = 12.70$.

Sometimes the answer to a specific problem may involve inverse reasoning.

Example 3. The pH of a given solution is 10.5; what is the hydrogen ion concentration?

Solution. $pH = -\log [H^+]; [H^+] = 10^{-10.5}$

$$\text{or} \quad [H^+] = 10^{-11} \times 10^{0.5} = 3.2 \times 10^{-11}.$$

Consider a problem with more direct pharmaceutical application.

Example 4. Normal gastric acidity in adult males is given as pH = 1.92. Assuming that this value is due entirely to secreted hydrochloric acid, how much HCl is present in 50.00 ml. of normal male gastric juice?

Solution.

$$pH = 1.92 = -\log [H^+] = 10^{-1.92}$$

$$[H] = [HCl] = 10^{-2} \times 10^{0.08}$$

$$= 1.2 \times 10^{-2} \text{ mole/L.} = 0.06 \times 10^{-2} \text{ mole/50 ml.}$$

$$1 \text{ mole HCl} = 36.46 \text{ gm.}; 36.46 \times 0.06 \times 10^{-2} = 0.0219 \text{ gm. HCl/50.0 ml.}$$

This problem might have been phrased in another way.

Example 5. It is required that a patient with achlorhydria adjust his gastric acidity to pH of 1.62 by taking dilute hydrochloric acid. The prescription calls for 5 ml. of 3.0 M HCl to be taken in one-half glass of water (125 ml.) after meals. Is this correct?

Solution.

$$5 \text{ ml.} \times 3.0 \text{ M} = 15 \text{ mM./125 ml.} = 120 \text{ mM./L.} = 12 \times 10^{-2} \text{ M}$$

$$\text{and} \quad pH = -\log [H^+] = -\log [12 \times 10^{-2}] = 2.00 - 1.08 = 0.92$$

This is considerably lower than required.

Example 6. We might now consider a very dilute solution of an acid, e.g., HCl 10^{-7} M. What would be the pH of such a solution? Clearly, because it is completely ionized, the HCl will yield 10^{-7} mole of H^+ to the solution, and at this concentration we might expect some contribution of H^+ from the ionization of water. How much? We know that for water $[H^+][OH^-] = 10^{-14}$ and that in this present case of very dilute HCl the $[H^+]$ is 10^{-7} *plus* some unknown amount (x) from the water.

Solution. We may write

$$(10^{-7} + x)(x) = 10^{-14} \text{ or } x^2 + 10^{-7}x - 10^{-14} = 0$$

Such quadratic equations may be solved by the general expression:

$$x = \frac{-b \pm \sqrt{b^2 - 4ac}}{2a}$$

where a and b are the coefficients of x^2 and x respectively and c is the third term in the expression. The answer, 6.15×10^{-8}, represents the amount of H^+ furnished by the ionization of water; 1×10^{-7} came from the HCl, so that the total $[H^+]$ is the sum of these or 1.62×10^{-7}. The pH = 6.79. At first glance we might have assumed that the pH would equal 7.00; why is it less?

Here, the H^+ from the HCl actually represses the ionization of water so that it does not contribute the same amount of H^+ (and OH^-) it would if it were pure (6.15×10^{-8} rather than 10^{-7}). This repression of the ionization by an ion common to both of the substances in solution is called the *common ion effect.*

WEAK ACIDS AND BASES

Weak acids and bases are a different matter; by definition they are weakly ionized and hence do not contribute their full complement of H^+ or OH^- to solutions. Consider acetic acid which has $K_i = 1.75 \times 10^{-5}$. It ionizes as follows:

$$CH_3COOH \leftrightarrows CH_3COO^- + H^+$$

which we might abbreviate to:

$$HOAc \leftrightarrows H^+ + OAc^-$$

and $K_{eq} = K_i = K_a = [H^+][OAc^-]/[HOAc] = 1.75 \times 10^{-5}$. For every mole of HOAc in solution we get something less than 1 mole—call it x—of H^+ and an equal amount of OAc^- leaving $1 - x$ mole of unionized HOAc in solution. Then:

$$K_a = [x][x]/[1 - x]$$

$$= 1.75 \times 10^{-5}$$

$$\text{or} \qquad x^2 + 1.75 \times 10^{-5}x - 1.75 \times 10^{-5} = 0$$

By application of the methods for the solution of quadratic equations we might solve for x; but if this is small compared to the concentration of the acid present, and it usually is, we might neglect it in the denominator without a great loss of accuracy, so that

$$x^2 = 1.75 \times 10^{-5} \text{ and } x = [H^+];$$

$$x = 4.18 \times 10^{-3} \text{ and } pH = 2.38$$

Go through these calculations and see if you agree.

Similar considerations apply to weak bases. Calculate for yourselves the pH of a 1 M solution of ammonium hydroxide whose K_b is 1.75×10^{-5}. Decide, also, which is the stronger acid, benzoic with $K_a = 6.3 \times 10^{-5}$ or salicylic with $K_a = 1.0 \times 10^{-3}$.

We come now to consider the *salts of weak acids (or bases).* These have some special properties. Sodium acetate is an example. It ionizes as follows:

$$NaOAc \leftrightarrows Na^+ + OAc^-$$

In aqueous solution, the acetate ion is able to accept a proton from water (functioning as an acid) thus behaving as a base. The acetic acid which is formed is, as we have seen, but weakly dissociated and some OH^- is formed thus conferring a degree of basicity to the solution.

Eq. 1 $$OAc^- + H_2O \leftrightarrows HOAc + OH^-$$

Applying equilibrium considerations to this system we have

Eq. 2 $$K_b = [HOAc]\,[OH^-]/[OAc^-]\,[H_2O]$$

In aqueous solution $[H_2O]$ can be neglected and since $K_aK_b = K_w$ it follows that

Eq. 3 $$K_w/K_a = [HOAc]\,[OH^-]/[OAc^-]$$

Given, then, a solution 0.1 M in sodium acetate, and K_a for acetic acid $= 1.85 \times 10^{-5}$, what is the pH of an aqueous solution of the salt? In other words, to what extent is the reaction represented by Equation 1 taking place, i.e., what is the $[OH^-]$ produced in the solution? The concentration of OH^-, which is equal to the concentration of HOAc formed, is the unknown quantity, x; $[OAc^-]$ will be $0.1 - x$, but since x will be small compared to 0.1 M, we will ignore it in this expression, so that substituting in Equation 3, we arrive at:

$$x^2/0.1 = K_w/K_a = 10^{-14}/1.75 \times 10^{-5}$$
$$x^2 = 10^{-14} \times 0.1/1.75 \times 10^{-5}$$
$$x = 7.5 \times 10^{-6} = [OH^-]$$
$$\text{pOH} = 5.12 \text{ and pH} = 8.88$$

The same considerations apply to the salts of strong acids and weak bases. Work out for yourselves the application of these principles to a solution of ammonium chloride.

BUFFERS

These concepts are the basis for a discussion of an important class of solutions called *buffers*. These are mixtures of a weak acid and one of its salts (or a weak base and one of its salts) which resist a change in pH when a small amount of acid (or base) is added to them. A familiar example is blood which, in normal health, maintains a pH between 7.40 and 7.45. You can appreciate the importance of pH with respect to the use of intravenous drugs or solutions which, obviously, cannot be permitted to make appreciable changes in this value. Furthermore, drugs to be given intravenously must be designed to accommodate to this pH range of blood since the forms in which they will be soluble, transported, and available to a specific receptor site will depend, in part, on this factor.

To develop this discussion, assume any weak acid, e.g., acetic acid. The following relationships should now be familiar:

$$K_a = [H^+]\,[OAc^-]/[HOAc]$$
$$[H^+] = K_a[HOAc]/[OAc^-]$$
$$-\log [H^+] = -\log K_a - \log [HOAc]/[OAc^-]$$
$$\text{pH} = \text{p}K_a - \log [HOAc]/[OAc^-]$$
$$\text{pH} = \text{p}K_a + \log [OAc^-]/[HOAc]$$

In other words, the pH in any such buffered solution is equal to the $\text{p}K_a$ + log [ionized form]/[unionized form]. The equation expressing the relationship between pH and pK is known as the *Henderson-Hasselbalch equation;* this simple modification of this equation will become quite familiar to us as we learn to apply it to a number of pharmaceutical problems.

Let's take a closer look at how these buffer solutions work. If we were to add 1 ml. of 0.1 M HCl to 99 ml. of pure water, the pH of the solution would be 3.00 (Are you convinced that this is so?). Suppose, instead, we were to add the HCl to 99 ml. of a mixture of acetic acid and sodium acetate 0.2 M in each. The pH of the buffer mixture is easy to determine:

$$pH = pK_a + \log [OAc^-]/[HOAc]$$

$$K_a = 1.75 \times 10^{-5}$$

$$pH = pK_a = 4.757$$

Now if we add 1 ml. of 0.1 M HCl, the H^+ therefrom can react with the OAc^- available from the sodium acetate to form undissociated acetic acid, thereby decreasing the quantity of OAc^- and increasing the quantity of HOAc in the mixture. We started with 99 ml. $\times$ 0.2 M = 19.8 mM. of OAc^-. We add $1 \times 0.1 = 0.1$ mM. of H^+ which reacts with OAc^- leaving 19.7 mM. and giving 19.9 mM. of acetic acid. Putting these new values into the equation,

$$pH = 4.757 + \log 19.7/19.9 = 4.767$$

Thus, by adding some strong acid to the buffer system, we have changed the pH only 0.010 units. Notice that in this case we have substituted the values for the actual number of millimoles present in 100 ml. of solution rather than converting to moles/liter as usually called for in the concentration terms in these equations. But remember that millimoles/milliliter equals moles/liter.

We have already referred to the blood as an effective buffer system. There are several contributors to the overall buffer capacity of the blood and among these is the carbonic acid-bicarbonate system.

$$CO_2 + H_2O \leftrightharpoons H_2CO_3 \leftrightharpoons H^+ + HCO_3^-$$

Applying the Henderson-Hasselbalch equation, we see that

$$pH = pK_a + \log [HCO_3^-]/[H_2CO_3].$$

Although pK_a for carbonic acid may be found in most texts or handbooks as 6.4, this applies to simple aqueous solutions. The same "constant" determined for the complex mixture which is blood is 6.1. The normal bicarbonate-carbonic acid ratio for blood is about 20:1. Substituting these values into the equation, it is clear that the pH of the blood is 7.4. This may change in diseases producing alkalosis (duodenal ulcer, pH = 7.5) or acidosis (diabetes, pH = 7.1). In acute diabetic acidosis, the pH of venous blood may drop as low as 6.9, but generally changes beyond ± 0.3 are considered extreme.

APPLICATION OF ACID-BASE THEORY

Having learned something of the theory of acids and bases, let's examine one or two specific examples of its use in laboratory practice. It is simple enough to say that in order to determine the amount of H^+ or OH^- yielded to a solution, it is only necessary to neutralize this H^+ or OH^- with some standard base (or acid) of known concentration. How do we do this? Since its concentration must be known accurately, the acid or base must be stable, easily dried and weighed, and reasonably soluble in water. Bases such as NaOH and KOH are not well suited to this purpose. They are hygroscopic, i.e., they absorb water from the air, and are therefore difficult to weigh and transfer. They also absorb CO_2 to form the carbonate ion, and for this reason even the water used in the preparation of their aqueous solutions should be boiled to remove this dissolved gas. After preparation, the solutions should be protected from the air to avoid subsequent conversion to carbonate during use. Observing these precautions, sodium hydroxide is often used as a *secondary standard* having been previously standardized against a standard acid. Most often this standard acid is potassium acid phthalate (KHP). It is a moderately strong acid ($K_a = 1.2 \times 10^{-3}$), mol.

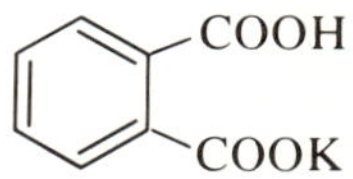

wt. = 204.23, and yields 1 mole of H^+ per mole. It is easily dried and weighed. If we were to weigh out 2.0423 gm. and dissolve this in 1 L. of water, the solution would be 0.010 M = 0.010 N. Having prepared a solution of sodium hydroxide of approximately this normality, it is only necessary to titrate a portion of the acid solution (e.g., 25.00 ml.) with base, record the amount of base used (e.g., 23.50 ml.), and calculate the normality of the base solution using the familiar expression:

$$\text{ml.}_{acid} \times N_{acid} = \text{ml.}_{base} \times N_{base};$$
$$25.00 \times 0.010 = 23.50 \times x$$
$$x = 0.011\ \text{N}$$

The sodium hydroxide may be used now, with the precautions cited above, to titrate other acids of unknown strength. You will have occasion to do this in the laboratory. The equivalence point in such a titration is reached when all of the H^+ has reacted with the OH^- to form water.

One of the commonly used methods for determining this point—we will consider other methods later—is by indicators. These are substances, generally organic dyes, which have one color (or may be colorless) at one pH and a different color at another. They behave just like the weak acids and bases we have discussed.

$$\text{HIn} \leftrightharpoons H^+ + \text{In}^-$$

and $$\text{pH} = \text{p}K_a + \log [\text{In}^-]/[\text{HIn}].$$

The sensitivity of our eyes is such that we can observe a distinct color change when the ratio of $[\text{In}^-]$ to [HIn] changes from approximately 1/10 to 10/1. Thus, the color change of the indicator will take place through the range pH = ±1. In any particular titration, an indicator is chosen which will change color over the expected range from immediately before to immediately after the equivalence point. This point is called the *equivalence point* rather than the neutral point because, as we have seen, the neutralization of a weak acid with a strong base results in the formation of the salt of the weak acid which, in solution, has a pH other than neutral (7.00). Suppose we were to titrate a weak acid like nicotinic acid which you may do in the laboratory. What would be the pH at the equivalence point if K_a =1.4

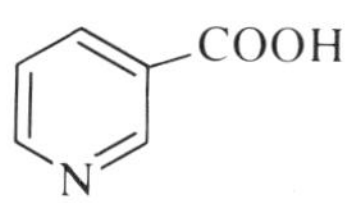

$\times 10^{-5}$ and mol. wt. = 123? Titration with sodium hydroxide will produce sodium nicotinate according to the following equation:

Eq. 4 $$RCOOH + NaOH \leftrightharpoons RCOONa + H_2O$$

When equilibrium is established, we end up with a solution of a salt of a weak acid and a strong base analogous to the sodium acetate case we discussed earlier. The nicotinate ion, acting as a base, can accept a proton from water to form undissociated nicotinic acid

Eq. 5 $$RCOO^- + H_2O \leftrightharpoons RCOOH + OH^-$$

Eq. 6 $$K_b = [RCOOH]\,[OH^-]/[RCOO^-] = K_w/K_a$$

Had we taken 25.0 ml. of a 0.1 M nicotinic acid solution to start with (2.5 mM.), added 25 ml. of water prior to titration, and used 25.0 ml. of 0.1 M NaOH for the titration, we would have produced according to Equation 4 2.5 mM. of nicotinate in a total volume of 75 ml. This corresponds to 33.3 mM./L. or 3.3×10^{-2} M. However, we do not yet know the extent of the reaction represented by Equation 5 except that $[RCOOH] = [OH^-] = x$. Therefore,

$$K_b = K_w/K_a = 1 \times 10^{-14}/1.4 \times 10^{-5} = 7.15 \times 10^{-10}$$

$$K_b = x^2/3.3 \times 10^{-2}$$

and since $$x = [OH^-] = 4.88 \times 10^{-6}$$

$$pOH = 5.31 \quad \text{and} \quad pH = 8.69$$

Similarly, with a weak base and a strong acid we can show that

Eq. 7 $$NH_3 + HCl \leftrightharpoons NH_4^+ + Cl^-$$

Eq. 8 $$NH_4^+ + H_2O \leftrightharpoons NH_4OH + H^+$$

Eq. 9 $$K_w/K_b = 10^{-14}/1.75 \times 10^{-5} = x^2/[NH_4^+]$$

If we were to titrate 25.0 ml. of 0.1 M NH_4OH with 25.0 ml. of 0.1 M HCl, show that the pH at the equivalence point would be 5.28.

In concluding our discussion of acid-base reactions, it is appropriate to mention titrations in nonaqueous media. Because of the weak basicity or acidity of many drug products and/or their poor water solubility, nonaqueous titration methods were developed for a large number of drugs in the decade between 1940 and 1950. A sampling from the U.S.P. shows that almost 25 percent of the assays now involve nonaqueous titrations, while aqueous titrations make up only 10 percent. Nonaqueous titrations have the same advantages of simplicity, speed, and accuracy as do aqueous methods. Their use eliminates the potential for competition between the drug of interest and water which may behave either as an acid or a base. For example, when a solution of a weak base is titrated with an aqueous perchloric acid solution, the following occurs:

$$RNH_2 + H_2O \rightleftharpoons RNH_3^+ + OH^-$$
$$HClO_4 + H_2O \rightleftharpoons H_3O^+ + ClO_4^-$$

The overall reaction is simply the formation of water:

$$H_3O^+ + OH^- \rightleftharpoons 2\,H_2O$$

If the equilibrium of the first reaction lies far to the left, a sharp end-point will not be observed for this titration. However, nonaqueous conditions may be chosen to eliminate these interactions with the solvent such that the perchloric acid would react directly with the amine resulting in a sharp end-point:

$$RNH_2 + HClO_4 \rightleftharpoons RNH_3^+ + ClO_4^-$$

The solvents used for nonaqueous titrations include methanol, acetic acid, acetic anhydride, chloroform, benzene, and dioxane, to name a few. Many of the U.S.P. procedures utilize acetic acid as the solvent. It undergoes the following reactions:

$$CH_3COOH + RNH_2 \rightleftharpoons RNH_3^+ + CH_3COO^-$$
$$CH_3COOH + HClO_4 \rightleftharpoons (CH_3COOH_2)^+\,ClO_4^-$$
$$(CH_3COOH_2)^+ + CH_3COO^- \rightleftharpoons 2\,CH_3COOH$$

Perchloric acid and hydrogen bromide in acetic acid are the common acids used when basic agents are assayed while acidic agents are normally titrated against standard solutions of sodium or lithium methoxide. Potassium methoxide is not used since it often forms a gelatinous reaction product. Precautions must be taken to insure that anhydrous conditions are maintained during the assay because even a trace amount of water will interfere. The end-points of nonaqueous titrations may be determined with either indicators or potentiometric methods. Examples of indicators which may be used include azoviolet, crystal violet, malachite green, and thymol blue. An example of a titration of this type is provided by the U.S.P. assay of phenytoin (diphenylhydantoin) which behaves as a weak acid.

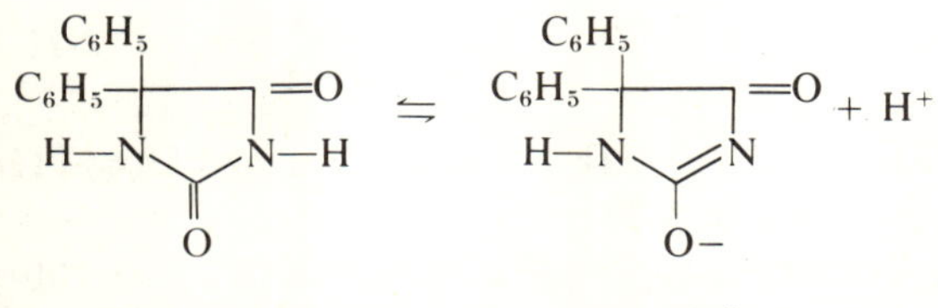

It is titrated in an anhydrous solvent (dimethylformamide) using sodium methoxide as the titrant (U.S.P. XIX, 379).

THINGS TO REMEMBER

$$\text{If } nA + mB \rightleftharpoons xC + yD$$

$$K_{eq} = \frac{[C]^x\,[D]^y}{[A]^n\,[B]^m}$$

$$pK_w = pH + pOH = 14$$

$$pH = \log \quad 1/[H^+] = -\log [H^+]$$

$$pH = pK_a + \log [A^-]/[HA]$$

Experiment 2. Standardization of Sodium Hydroxide Solution

A solution of approximately 1.0 N sodium hydroxide will be prepared for your use.

Accurately weigh three portions of approximately 5 gm. each of dry potassium acid phthalate ($C_8H_5O_4K$, mol. wt. 204.23). Transfer each 5-gm. portion to individual 250 ml. Erlenmeyer flasks and add about 100 ml. of distilled water (graduated cylinder). Use small portions of water to wash any powder remaining in the weighing bottle into the flask. When the substance has completely dissolved, add a drop or two of phenolphthalein indicator and titrate with the sodium hydroxide solution, from a previously filled buret, until the color is a faint persistent pink. If you have any doubt that you have reached the end-point, record the buret reading and add one more drop (0.05 ml.) of the NaOH solution.

Compute the normality of the NaOH solution as follows: from the weight of the KHP calculate the number of milliequivalents in each of the three samples. Then

$$\text{Normality} = \text{mEq./ml. used in the titration}$$

Record the mean value of the three determinations on the label of your NaOH bottle. Reserve it for future experiments. Keep the bottle tightly capped when not in use.

> NOTE: Before the end of the laboratory period remove the stopcock from your buret, wash the buret thoroughly including the stopcock and barrel, and return it to your equipment drawer clean and dry.

Experiment 3. Boric Acid Assay

Boric acid acts as a very weak monobasic acid:

$$H_3BO_3 \leftrightharpoons H^+ + BO_2^- + H_2O$$

Long before an equivalent amount of sodium hydroxide has been added to neutralize it, the reaction is forced to the left and a change in the color of the phenolphthalein indicator occurs. However, if glycerin is added to the titration mixture, it forms a slightly dissociated complex with the metaborate ion (BO_2^-) thus preventing this reversal.

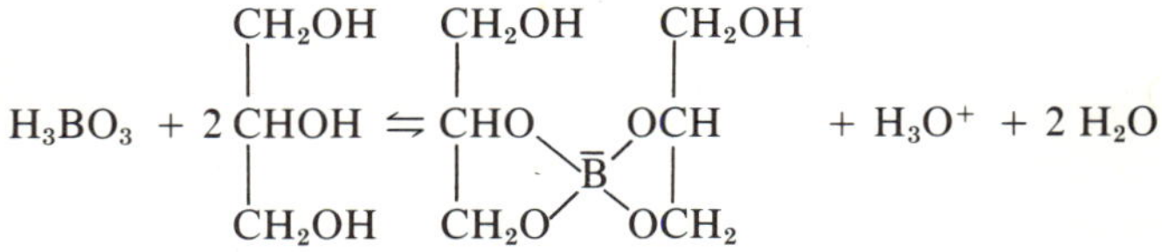

As a result, the pH during the titration remains below 8 until an equivalent of sodium hydroxide has been added.

1. Rinse out a clean buret once or twice with small portions of standard sodium

hydroxide (1.0 N) solution. Allow the buret to drain and discard the washings. Fill it to the zero mark.

2. Transfer 200 ml. of glycerin to a beaker. Add a few drops of phenolphthalein indicator and sufficient NaOH solution (a few drops) to bring the glycerin to the indicator end-point (light pink). Use a stirring rod to insure good mixing.

3. With a pipet transfer 25.0 ml. of your unknown boric acid solution to an Erlenmeyer flask. Using a graduated cylinder, add 30 ml. of the neutralized glycerin and a few drops of indicator. Swirl the flask to mix the solutions thoroughly.

4. Record the buret reading. Titrate the mixture to the end-point with NaOH. Again add 25 ml. of neutralized glycerin and if the pink color is discharged, continue the titration until it reappears. Record the volume of the NaOH used.

5. Repeat the titration with two additional samples of your boric acid solution.

6. Calculate the concentration of boric acid in your samples; express the result in grams per 100 ml.

7. Clean and dry your buret thoroughly, including the stopcock, before returning your equipment to the drawer.

Experiment 4. Phenytoin Assay

Phenytoin ($C_{15}H_{12}N_2O_2$) is a white powder, practically insoluble in water. Using a weighing bottle, weigh accurately a sample of about 500 mg. of the dried powder provided. Transfer it quantitatively to an Erlenmeyer flask. Dissolve it in 50 ml. (graduated cylinder) of anhydrous dimethylformamide using small portions of the solvent to wash out any small amounts of powder adhering to the weighing bottle. Add three drops of azoviolet indicator and titrate the sample with 0.10 N sodium methoxide solution to the appearance of a blue color.

Repeat the titration using two additional samples of phenytoin and a blank of 50 ml. of dimethylformamide alone, making any necessary correction to your titration of the samples.

Calculations for nonaqueous titrations are identical to those used in titrimetry in general:

$$\text{ml.} \times \text{N} = \text{mEq.}$$

$$\text{mEq.} \times \text{mEq. wt.} = \text{milligrams}$$

$$\frac{\text{mg. assayed}}{\text{mg. sample}} \times 100 = \text{percent purity}$$

Calculate the mean percent purity of your phenytoin sample.

PROBLEMS

1. Define the following terms: (a) normality, (b) molarity, (c) milliequivalent, (d) equivalent, (e) equivalent weight.
2. Calculate the normality of each of the following solutions:
   (a) 10 percent w/v sulfuric acid
   (b) sodium hydroxide solution 40.00 ml. of which is equivalent to 0.7500 gm. of potassium acid phthalate.
3. A solution of sulfuric acid was standardized using pure sodium carbonate, 25.00 ml.

being used to completely neutralize 0.3100 gm. of the latter. The sulfuric acid was then used to titrate 25.00 ml. of a sodium hydroxide solution of unknown strength, 35.00 ml. being used. What was the normality of the sodium hydroxide?

4. What is the pH of the final solution obtained when 40.0 ml. of 0.10 M HCl is added to 80.0 ml. of 0.2 M NaOH?
5. If 25 ml. of 0.200 M acetic acid are diluted to 50.0 ml. and titrated with 0.100 M NaOH, find the pH when half of the acid has been neutralized ($K_a = 1.75 \times 10^{-5}$).
6. When 200 ml. of 0.0010 M NaOH are added to 300 ml. of 0.00050 M HCl, what is the pH of the solution?
7. How many grams of sodium acetate must be added to 300 ml. of 0.100 M acetic acid to produce a buffer with a pH of 6.50?
8. What is the pH of a buffer which has been prepared by mixing 250 mg. of ammonium chloride and 200 ml. of 0.100 M ammonia solution?
   What is the pH of this mixture after 10 mM. of HCl has been added? The addition of the acid dilutes the mixture to 250 ml.
9. If 50 ml. of 0.100 M ammonia is mixed with 100 ml. of 0.100 M HCl, what is the pH of the resulting mixture?
10. Find the H_3O^+ concentrations which correspond to the following values: (a) pH = 8.95, (b) pH = 3.85, (c) pOH = 4.50, (d) pOH = 0.30.
11. As a hospital pharmacist you are asked to prepare and analyze 2 ml. vials containing 50 mg./ml. of Meperidine Hydrochloride Injection. After preparation of the solution, you carry out the U.S.P. assay which involves extraction of the free base followed by a nonaqueous titration with perchloric acid. If a series of 1 ml. samples required an average of 1.90 ml. of 0.100 N perchloric acid for titration, how much drug was present per vial? (Meperidine hydrochloride = $C_{15}H_{22}NO_2Cl$.)
12. A 365 mg. sample of succinylcholine chloride was placed in glacial acetic acid and titrated with 0.100 M perchloric acid. Determine the percent purity of the salt if 20.00 ml. of $HClO_4$ solution was required to reach the end-point. (Succinylcholine chloride = $C_{14}H_{30}N_2O_4Cl_2$.)

ANSWERS

2. (a) 2.04 N
   (b) 0.09180 N
3. 0.3276 N
4. 13.0
5. 4.76
6. 10
7. 140
8. 9.88, 9.08
9. 1.48
10. (a) 1.1×10^{-9}
    (b) 1.4×10^{-4}
    (c) 3.1×10^{-10}
    (d) 1.9×10^{-14}
11. 108 mg.
12. 99.0 percent

Chapter 4

Precipitation Reactions—Solubility Product

You will recall our earlier mention of reactions which are almost wholly irreversible (p. 19), i.e., those in which the equilibrium lies almost completely in one direction. Examples were the reactions leading to the formation of a gas or of an insoluble substance, in which the component atoms or ions are effectively removed from the mixture and any appreciable reversal of the reaction is prevented. It is easy to see, then, that such reactions can be useful for certain quantitative estimations. If an insoluble product results, it might simply be removed by filtration, washed, dried, and weighed. Indeed, methods for the determination of chloride in injectables, biological fluids, sea water, and similar solutions, and of sulfate, iron, and many other ions, have been based on this simple procedure. It must be recognized, however, that these "insoluble" substances are not *completely* insoluble; some molecules, depending on circumstances, will dissolve to yield ions to the solution. These will result in the establishment of an equilibrium which can be described as follows:

$$AB_{solid} \leftrightarrows AB_{solution} \leftrightarrows A^+ + B^-$$

As for any other equilibrium,

$$\frac{[A^+][B^-]}{[AB]_{solution}} = \text{constant (k).}$$

Because the amount of AB in solution is constant, we can combine this term with k to give the following expression:

$$[A^+][B^-] = K_{sp}$$

This is called the *solubility product constant,* sometimes designated *S*, and is constant for a given solute, solvent, and temperature. To complete the derivation of the expression we must, as we did with K_{eq}, raise each term to the power represented by the number of ions or molecules entering into the reaction. Thus, if

$$A_mB_n \leftrightarrows mA^{n+} + nB^{m-}$$

then $$K_{sp} = [A^{n+}]^m [B^{m-}]^n$$

Here are a few examples:

$$Ag^+ + Cl^- \leftrightarrows AgCl \quad ; K_{sp} = [Ag^+][Cl^-]$$

$$Pb^{2+} + 2\,Cl^- \leftrightarrows PbCl_2 \quad ; K_{sp} = [Pb^{2+}][Cl^-]^2$$

$$Fe^{3+} + 3\,OH^- \leftrightarrows Fe(OH)_3 \quad ; K_{sp} = [Fe^{3+}][OH^-]^3$$

$$2\,Bi^{3+} + 3\,S^= \leftrightarrows Bi_2S_3 \quad ; K_{sp} = [Bi^{3+}]^2[S^=]^3$$

You will find a table of commonly used solubility product constants in the appendix.

In addition to the separation of ions from solution by precipitation, this principle might be invoked to determine the residual solubility of insoluble substances or the pH of suspensions of insoluble inorganic precipitates. Calcium Hydroxide Solution (U.S.P. XIX, 63) is a saturated solution of $Ca(OH)_2$ in water; the liquid is dispensed as an astringent. How much $Ca(OH)_2$ does this contain? If the K_{sp} for calcium hydroxide is 4×10^{-5}, and $Ca(OH)_2 \leftrightarrows Ca^{++} + 2\,OH^-$, then

$$[Ca^{++}][OH^-]^2 = 4 \times 10^{-5}$$

$$x \times (2x)^2 = 4 \times 10^{-5}$$

and $x = [Ca^{++}] = [Ca(OH)_2] = 2.16 \times 10^{-2}$ moles/L. The formula weight of calcium hydroxide is 74; $74 \times 2.16 \times 10^{-2} = 1.60$ gm./L. What is the pH of such a solution? $[OH^-] = 2[Ca^{++}] = 4.32 \times 10^{-2}$ M; pOH = 1.36 and pH = 12.6.

Generally speaking, most difficulty with solubility product problems involves the decision as to when and when not to multiply a given concentration before raising it to the appropriate power called for in the equation. Consider the reaction

$$Fe(OH)_3 \leftrightarrows Fe^{3+} + 3\,OH^-$$

Keep in mind the definitions we have established for problems of this type; remember that [ ] indicates molar concentration and that

$$K_{sp} = [A^{n+}]^m [B^{m-}]^n.$$

If K_{sp} is given and the concentration of either one of the ions is called for, it should be clear that if $[Fe^{3+}] = x$, then $[OH^-] = 3x$. Or should you decide to let $[OH^-] = x$, then $[Fe^{3+}] = x/3$.

$$x \times 27x^3 = K_{sp}$$

$$\text{or} \qquad (x/3) \times x^3 = K_{sp}.$$

If, on the other hand, one of the ion concentrations is given, the question asked is: "What is the concentration of the other?"

Example 1. $Fe(OH)_3$ is to be precipitated in an excess (0.1 M) of OH^-. What is the amount of Fe^{3+} (or $Fe(OH)_3$) which will remain unprecipitated? $K_{sp} = 1.1 \times 10^{-36}$.

Solution. Since $[OH^-] = 0.1$ M and $[Fe^{3+}] = [Fe(OH)_3]$

$$(0.1)^3x = K_{sp}$$

$$x = K_{sp}/0.001 = 1.1 \times 10^{-33} \text{ moles/L.}$$

Example 2. If 0.01 M Fe^{3+} is to be precipitated with OH^-, what concentration of the latter will be required?

Solution. In this case, $[Fe^{3+}] = 0.01$ and $[OH^-] = x$, so that $0.01x^3 = K_{sp}$ and $x = \sqrt[3]{K_{sp}/0.01} = \sqrt[3]{1.1 \times 10^{-34}} = 4.71 \times 10^{-12}$ moles/L.

There are a couple of other important effects we must consider in the application of these principles to analytical problems. One of these is the familiar common ion effect. Suppose we were to precipitate Ag^+ as $AgIO_3$ using 0.1 M (excess) of $NaIO_3$; how will the concentration of Ag^+ change? In pure water, the matter is simple:

$$Ag^+ + IO_3^- \leftrightharpoons AgIO_3$$

$$[Ag^+][IO_3^-] = K_{sp} = 3.1 \times 10^{-8}$$

$$[Ag^+] = 1.76 \times 10^{-4} \text{ M}$$

Now if an excess of IO_3^- is present, and $x = [Ag^+]$, then $[IO_3^-] = 0.1 + x$ and $x \times (0.1 + x) = 3.1 \times 10^{-8}$; x is small compared to 0.1 and we may simplify to $[Ag^+][0.1] = 3.1 \times 10^{-8}$ and $x = [Ag^+] = 3.1 \times 10^{-7}$ M. Thus there is a 1000-fold decrease in the solubility of $AgIO_3$ due to the presence of the excess of the iodate iron. For this reason, it is common practice to conduct these precipitation reactions with a slight excess of the precipitant to insure completeness of reaction.

Example 3. Barium Sulfate U.S.P. is used as a gastrointestinal radiopaque medium. How many milligrams will dissolve in 100 ml. of 0.1 M Na_2SO_4? $K_{sp} = 1.3 \times 10^{-10}$.

Solution. $[Ba^{++}][SO_4^=] = 1.3 \times 10^{-10}$; $x \times 0.1 = 1.3 \times 10^{-10}$

$$x = 13 \times 10^{-10} \text{ M} = 3.034 \times 10^{-4} \text{ mg./L.} = 3.034 \times 10^{-5} \text{ mg./100 ml.}$$

Another effect is that of the pH of the medium on the solubility of precipitates. Consider, for example, the effect of the presence of acid on the solubility of $PbSO_4$. In pure water, $Pb^{++} + SO_4^= \leftrightharpoons PbSO_4$. If an excess of H^+ were present, $H^+ + SO_4^= \leftrightharpoons HSO_4^-$. This ion is an acid ($K_i = 1.2 \times 10^{-2}$) which, because it is not completely ionized, has the net effect of removing $SO_4^=$, thus increasing the dissolution of $PbSO_4$ in order to resupply $SO_4^=$ and restore equilibrium. In other words, the solubility of lead sulfate is increased in an acid medium. Generally, any ion which is capable of acting as a conjugate base of a weak acid will behave similarly; acetate, oxalate, carbonate, phosphate, all can react with H^+ to form slightly ionized species. To overcome problems of this sort, precipitation may be carried out in buffered solution.

One way to avoid the complications of quantitative precipitation is by means of a *precipitation titration reaction* in which the precipitate is not isolated but in which the completeness of the precipitate's formation is indicated in some way that permits a titration for its determination. Consider, for example, the determination of chloride by the now familiar formation of silver chloride. If we were to titrate an unknown chloride solution with standard silver nitrate, it is clear that enough silver nitrate would be used to precipitate all of the Cl^-. How can we recognize the first drop of excess silver? From your previous experience, it is easy to guess: use an indicator which produces a color with Ag^+. Such an indicator is $CrO_4^=$, the chromate ion (yellow); Ag_2CrO_4 is a red precipitate. As Ag^+ is added to the solution, AgCl precipitates; and when all the Cl^- is used up, the first drop of excess Ag^+ precipitates the red chromate salt, thus indicating the end-point. Adsorption indicators may also be used; in the determination of Br^- with standard Ag^+, the dye eosin (red orange) is used. This dye is actually adsorbed on the surface of the particles of AgBr precipitate and changes in color to a reddish violet in the presence of excess silver.

Finally, some indicators form soluble colored complexes with an excess of the reagent. An example of this is seen in the assay of Sodium Chloride for Injection (U.S.P. XIX, 457) in which the Cl^- is wholly precipitated by an excess of Ag^+. This excess can now be titrated with a standard CNS^- solution inasmuch as it will also form an insoluble substance, AgCNS. Ferric ion is used as an indicator because the slightest excess of CNS^- will form the deep reddish brown $Fe(CNS)_3$. The excess Ag^+, subtracted from the total added initially, is an amount equivalent to the Cl^- present. Because AgCNS is less soluble than AgCl, one must guard against an excess of CNS^- for, as you now appreciate, $AgCl + CNS^- \leftrightarrows AgCNS + Cl^-$ which would put Cl^- back into solution leading to over-titration. In this particular procedure, some nitrobenzene is added to the titration mixture. This coats the particles of AgCl and helps prevent their dissolution.

PROBLEMS

1. Write the equilibrium reaction and the solubility product expression for the following: (a) PbS, (b) Ag_3PO_4, (c) $Fe(OH)_3$, (d) $AgIO_3$, (e) BaF_2.
2. Using the values for K_{sp} given in the appendix, calculate the following:
   (a) The molar solubility of PbS
   (b) The concentration of $PO_4^{\equiv}$ to be expected in pure water containing Ag_3PO_4
   (c) The ferric ion concentration of a suspension of ferric hydroxide in distilled water
   (d) The molar solubility of $AgIO_3$
   (e) The fluoride ion concentration remaining after an equivalent of barium ion has been added to a solution of fluoride ion and allowed to reach equilibrium
3. (a) In 2(e) above, what would be the solubility of the BaF_2 in 0.1 M NaF?
   (b) In 2(d), what is the Ag^+ concentration in 0.1 M $NaIO_3$?
   (c) In 2(c), what would be the effect of an excess of ammonium hydroxide used as the precipitant?
   (d) How many milligrams of Ag_3PO_4 will dissolve in 100 ml. of 0.1 M Na_3PO_4?
4. Outline an analytical procedure to determine the amounts of HCl and NaCl in a dilute aqueous solution containing both.
5. Milk of Magnesia (U.S.P. XIX, 291) is an 8 percent suspension of magnesium hydroxide [$Mg(OH)_2$] in water which is used as a laxative. How much $Mg(OH)_2$ is actually dissolved in 1 L.? Calculate the pH of such a suspension.
6. The classical determination of Mg^{++} involves its precipitation as magnesium ammonium phosphate, $MgNH_4PO_4$, for which $K_{sp} = 3.0 \times 10^{-13}$. How many milligrams of $MgSO_4$ would remain in 100 ml. of a solution from which $MgSO_4$ had been precipitated by 0.05 M $(NH_4)_3PO_4$?
7. Given a 0.02 M solution of Ag^+ and a solution 0.001 M in Pb^{++} and adding by drops a

concentrated solution of K_2CrO_4 (neglect any volume change), show by appropriate calculations which precipitate will form first.

ANSWERS

2. (a) 2.05×10^{-14}
   (b) 1.45×10^{-3}
   (c) 4.5×10^{-10}
   (d) 1.8×10^{-4}
   (e) 1.51×10^{-2}
3. (a) 1.7×10^{-4}
   (b) 3.1×10^{-7}
   (c) decreased solubility of $Fe(OH)_3$
   (d) 14.7 mg.
5. 11.9 mg./L., pH = 10.61
6. 4.81×10^{-5}
7. Pb^{++} requires 1.8×10^{-11} M/L. vs. 2.75×10^{-9} for Ag^+

Chapter 5

Complexometric Titrations

A third method by which an equilibrium may be shifted to essentially a quantitative, unidirectional reaction involves the formation of slightly dissociated but usually soluble complexes. As early as 1750 it was found that certain metals can react with neutral molecules, in stoichiometric proportions, to form complex compounds:

$$CoCl_3 + 6\,NH_3 \rightarrow \text{in air} \rightarrow Co(NH_3)_6Cl_3$$

The product, a bright orange-yellow crystalline substance, was salt-like in that the Cl was still ionic (could be precipitated with Ag^+) but the manner in which the NH_3 was included in the compound was not clear. We now know that in this case, as well as in many other metal-complex compounds, the NH_3 is bound not by ionic valence, nor by covalent bonds as in organic compounds, but by what has been called the *coordinate-covalent bond.* In this bond the free electron pairs of a neutral or an ionic species are donated to the metal atom.

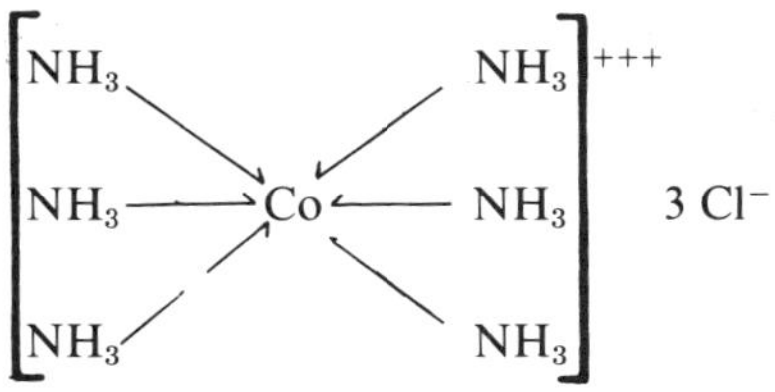

Metals vary in their ability to complex in this way. The number of electron pairs which can be accepted in this manner is called the *coordination number.* It varies from 2 to 8 and is most commonly from 4 to 6.

For our purposes it is sufficient to summarize this phenomenon in a few simple rules and definitions:

1. The donor atom (e.g., the N of NH_3) is usually nonmetallic and often part of a molecule capable of independent existence.
2. It may also be a negative or a positive ion such as NO_3^- or $N_2H_5^+$.
3. The donor ion or molecule is called a *ligand* or *chelating agent*.
4. The *complex* or *chelate* thus formed may be positively or negatively charged or neutral depending on the balance of the electron charge on the metal. It may be labile; a ligand

weakly held to the metal may be replaced with another ligand to form a more stable complex; or it may be inert, the ligand being tightly bound to the metal.

5. Ligands which are bound in a complex at only one point are called *unidentate,* e.g.:

$$Cu^{++} + NH_3 \rightharpoonup Cu(NH_3)^{++} \rightharpoonup Cu(NH_3)_2^{++} \rightharpoonup Cu(NH_3)_4^{++}$$

Others which offer two or more points of attachment are called *multidentate,* e.g.:

$$H_2N{-}CH_2{-}CH_2{-}NH_2$$

To use complex formation as an analytical tool, certain conditions must be met: (1) the reaction to form the complex must be rapid, (2) the stoichiometry must be well defined (in the copper-ammonia case cited above, mixtures may be formed), and (3) we must be able to determine the end-point. For example, the chromium ion hydrates in aqueous medium (most ions do this) to form hexaaquochromium, $Cr(H_2O)_6^{3+}$ which is violet. It reacts with CN^- to form $Cr(CN)_6^{\equiv}$ which is yellow. Conditions (2) and (3) are fulfilled, but CN^- replaces H_2O only with difficulty, the reaction is slow, and it is therefore not suited to titrimetry.

For general, all-around, analytical purposes the most useful ligand is probably ethylenediaminetetraacetic acid commonly known and referred to as EDTA.

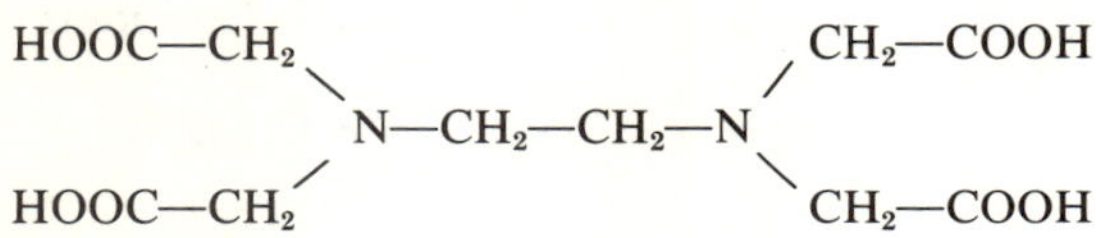

It has four electron pairs available for coordination at the oxygen atoms, and two more available at the nitrogen atoms. It forms chelates with nearly all metal ions. The reaction usually is rapid, the complexes are stable, and the stoichiometry is always 1:1.

EDTA is a tetraprotic acid, each step in the ionization of which has its own ionization constant. The dissociation and the concentration of each of the forms in solution are therefore pH-dependent, but note that it is not the salt-forming properties of EDTA which interest us at the moment, but its ability to form coordination complexes with metals. In fact, because of the low solubility of the acid itself in water, we most often use its disodium salt which undergoes the same reactions.

$$Na_2H_2Y \leftrightharpoons H_2Y^= + 2\,Na^+$$

$$Ca^{++} + H_2Y^= \leftrightharpoons CaY^= + 2\,H^+$$

As for any other equilibrium reaction we may write:

$$\frac{[CaY^=]\,[H^+]^2}{[Ca^{++}]\,[H_2Y^=]} = K$$

In this case, K is called the formation constant (K_f). Calculations can be made using this expression as with other equilibrium constants. Thus, if we know the pH (and this can be fixed with a buffer), the amount of free Ca^{++} remaining in solution can be calculated. If the pH is kept high (i.e., the H^+ concentration low), most of the Ca^{++} will be chelated and the equilibrium will lie far to the right. $CaY^=$ does not dissociate to any great extent; therefore the amount of $CaY^=$ formed is equal to the amount of Ca^{++} originally in solution.

The question at this point is: how do we determine the end-points in these titrations? The most common method is by the use of indicators which are themselves chelating agents and which form colored complexes with metal ions. Eriochrome black T is an example:

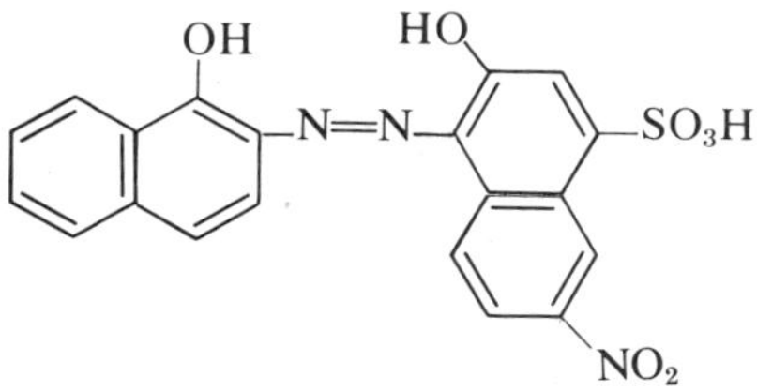

We can illustrate its use in the titration of magnesium by:

Eq. 1 $$\underset{}{Mg^{++}} + \underset{\text{(blue)}}{HIn^{=}} \leftrightharpoons \underset{\text{(red)}}{MgIn^{-}} + H^{+}$$

The K_f for the indicator complex must be smaller than that for the EDTA complex, and $MgIn^-$ must be sufficiently stable so that there is no reversal of the reaction before the end-point is reached. Thus, if we titrate with EDTA ($H_2Y^=$), the following represents what takes place:

Eq. 2 $$\underset{\text{(red)}}{MgIn^{-}} + H_2Y^{=} \leftrightharpoons MgY^{=} + \underset{\text{(blue)}}{HIn^{=}} + H^{+}$$

The ion content of the water used for these titrations is very important. Hard water which contains Ca^{++} and/or Mg^{++} cannot be used nor can water that has been delivered through copper pipes. Distilled or deionized water is required.

Some examples of the standardization and use of EDTA in the laboratory may be given. For standardization, one ordinarily uses calcium carbonate but for very precise work pure Zn (99.999 percent or greater) has been used. An amount of the metal, e.g., 0.3305 gm., is dissolved in dilute acid and the resulting solution is transferred quantitatively to a 500 ml. volumetric flask and made up to the mark. The solution contains 0.0101 moles/L. (Convince yourselves of this.). Portions of this solution (25.00 ml.) are then titrated with a solution of approximately 3.9 gm. $Na_2EDTA(2\ H_2O)$/L. Since the molarity of the Zn^{++} solution is known with accuracy and since milliliters $\times$ molarity = millimoles, the molarity of the EDTA solution is easily calculated.

The U.S.P. (XIX, 65) describes the assay of calcium pantothenate (mol. wt. = 476.54) by EDTA titration: 1 ml. 0.05 M EDTA = 0.05 mM. = 0.05 mM. Ca^{++}; total Ca^{++} = 0.05 $\times$ ml. EDTA used in the titration. Calcium carbonate and calcium gluconate are assayed in the same way.

An idea of the completeness of EDTA titrations and a comparison with solubility product methods can be had from computations such as the following:

Example. What is the concentration of Zn^{++} remaining in solution after titrating 50.0 ml. of 0.02 M zinc solution with 0.02 M EDTA at pH = 10?

Solution. $Zn^{++} + H_2Y^{=} \leftrightharpoons ZnY^{=} + 2\ H^{+}$, and K_f is given by:

$$\frac{[ZnY^{=}]\,[H^{+}]^2}{[H_2Y^{=}]\,[Zn^{++}]}$$

At equilibrium, $[ZnY^{=}] = 1/2\,[H^+]$ and $[H_2Y^{=}] = [Zn^{++}] = x$; if $K_f = 3.2 \times 10^{16}$ then:

$$3.2 \times 10^{16} = \frac{[10^{-10}]^2\,[0.5 \times 10^{-10}]}{x^2}$$

$$x = \sqrt{\frac{[10^{-20}]\,[0.5 \times 10^{-10}]}{3.2 \times 10^{16}}} = 3.95 \times 10^{-22} \text{ moles/L.}$$

This compares with $[Zn^{++}]$ = approximately 3.2×10^{-11} after precipitation as ZnS and the EDTA method is much more convenient and rapid.

Variations in the method are possible. To determine Mg^{++} in a solution of $MgCl_2$, one can do the following: An excess (50.0 ml.) of 0.022 M EDTA solution is added to 25.0 ml. of $MgCl_2$ solution. All of the Mg^{++} is complexed. The excess of EDTA is then titrated with 0.025 M Zn^{++} solution, 20.72 ml. being used. The strength of the $MgCl_2$ solution is calculated:

$$50.0 \times 0.022 = 1.10 \text{ mM. EDTA originally}$$

$$20.7 \times 0.025 = 0.518 \text{ mM. excess EDTA}$$

The difference, 0.582 mM., represents that used for the $MgCl_2$, and

$$\text{ml.} \times \text{M} = \text{mM.}; \quad 0.582/25.0 = 0.0233 \text{ M } MgCl_2$$

Similar considerations apply to the complexes formed in certain precipitation reactions. A reaction such as

$$Ag^+ + 2\,CN^- \leftrightarrows [Ag(CN)_2]^-$$

with $K_f = 1.26 \times 10^{21}$ can be used for the determination of cyanide or silver because, on addition of the first drop of excess Ag^+, $Ag[Ag(CN)_2]$ precipitates:

$$[Ag(CN)_2]^- + Ag^+ \leftrightarrows Ag[Ag(CN)_2].$$

Suppose, now, we had 110 ml. of $AgNO_3$ solution of unknown concentration. We add to this 300 ml. of 0.0200 M KCN (an excess) and titrate the excess with a silver nitrate solution of known concentration, e.g., 100.0 ml. of 0.015 M. What was the concentration of the original $AgNO_3$? A logical, stepwise approach to the problem is simplest. The equations covering the entire process may be written:

$$Ag^+ + 2\,CN^- \leftrightarrows [Ag(CN)_2]^-$$

$$Ag^+ + [Ag(CN)_2]^- \leftrightarrows Ag[Ag(CN)_2]$$

Now, the KCN is added; 0.02 M × 0.3 L. = 0.006 mole. The excess was 0.015 M × 0.1 L. = 0.0015 mole, measured by the standard Ag^+ solution used. Since $[Ag^+]$ used = $[CN^-]/2$, $[CN^-]$ = 0.0030 mole. We started with 0.006 mole; 0.006 − 0.003 = 0.003 mole of CN^- reacted with the original Ag^+ which must be 0.0015 mole. The original concentration was 0.0015 moles/0.11 L. = 0.0136 M.

There is still another way in which complex formation can be used for analytical determinations. Using the reaction

$$Ag^+ + 2\,NH_3 \leftrightharpoons [Ag(NH_3)_2]^+$$

a trace of iodide is added to form a little AgI, a solid, which makes the solution turbid and will serve as an end-point indicator. If we now titrate with a standard solution of CN^-,

$$[Ag(NH_3)_2]^+ + 2\,CN^- \leftrightharpoons [Ag(CN)_2]^- + 2\,NH_3$$

takes place because the cyanide complex is more stable than the ammonia complex. The AgI stays suspended in solution but finally, at the equivalence point, the CN^- reacts with the AgI

$$\underset{\text{(solid)}}{AgI} + 2\,CN^- \leftrightharpoons \underset{\text{(soluble)}}{[Ag(CN)_2]^-} + I^-$$

and the solution becomes clear. There are many modifications of these complexometric titrations which require a minimum of equipment and calculation.

Experiment 5. Magnesium Sulfate Solution for Injection Assay (U.S.P. XIX, 293)

Standardization of EDTA. Weigh out approximately 9.3 gm. of EDTA and quantitatively transfer the powder to a 400 ml. beaker containing 100 to 200 ml. of distilled water. Dissolve as much of the salt as possible, warming to 50°C. if necessary. (If you had prepared this solution during the preceding laboratory period, this step will not be necessary.) Cool and transfer the solution to a 500 ml. volumetric flask and adjust the volume to mark. Mix thoroughly and make sure all the solid is dissolved.

Weigh accurately about 200 mg. of calcium carbonate and transfer this quantitatively to a 400 ml. beaker. Add 10 ml. of distilled water and swirl to form a slurry. Introduce 2 ml. of dilute (10 percent) hydrochloric acid. Swirl the contents of the beaker to dissolve the calcium carbonate. Wash down the sides of the beaker with distilled water to make about 100 ml. While stirring add about 30 ml. of EDTA solution from a 50 ml. buret. Add 15 ml. of a 4 percent sodium hydroxide solution and 300 mg. of hydroxynaphthol blue indicator. Continue the titration with the EDTA solution to a blue end-point. The molarity of the EDTA solution can be calculated as follows:

$$M = \frac{\text{mg. } CaCO_3}{100.09 \times \text{ml. EDTA}}$$

Analysis of $MgSO_4$ Solution. Transfer 25.0 ml. (by pipet) of your unknown solution to each of three Erlenmeyer flasks and dilute with distilled water to about 100 ml. Using a dropper, adjust the pH of the solution to about 7 (use pH paper) with 4 percent sodium hydroxide, add 5 ml. of ammonia-ammonium chloride buffer solution (use a graduated cylinder, NOT a pipet) and 50 mg. of eriochrome black T indicator. Titrate with EDTA solution to a blue end-point. Calculate the concentration of $MgSO_4$ in your unknown and express the results as the mean of the three determinations in terms of grams of $MgSO_4$ (7 H_2O)/100 ml.

PROBLEMS

1. Zinc chloride, an astringent and dentin desensitizer, is assayed by titration with EDTA (U.S.P. XIX, 542). A sample of $ZnCl_2$ weighing 11.50 gm. was dissolved in water and made up to 1000 ml. Then, 25 ml. of this solution was diluted with water and titrated with 0.0500 M EDTA solution, 17.00 ml. of the EDTA solution being used. How pure was the $ZnCl_2$?
2. A sample of 10.00 ml. of an assay preparation of Alumina and Magnesia Oral Suspension (U.S.P. XIX, 19) required 10.00 ml. of 0.0500 M EDTA for determination of $Mg(OH)_2$ by titration. What was the concentration in milligrams per 10 ml. of $Mg(OH)_2$ in the sample, assuming that under the conditions of the assay only that substance was titrated?
3. Aluminum Hydroxide Gel (U.S.P. XIX, 21) is a well-known antacid which is analyzed by titration with EDTA. Twenty ml. of a solution of $Al(OH)_3$ dissolved in HCl required 30.85 ml. of 0.0500 M EDTA for titration. This corresponds to how much Al_2O_3 in the sample?
4. A sample of dry silver nitrate weighing 0.685 gm. was dissolved in 50 ml. of water. Following acidification of the solution with 2 ml. of nitric acid and addition of 2 ml. of ferric ammonium sulfate solution, the mixture was titrated using 0.1000 N NH_4CNS. If the $AgNO_3$ was 100 percent pure, how many milliliters were used (U.S.P. XIX, 451)?
5. A sample of zinc nitrate (15.0 ml.) required 21.0 ml. of 0.45 M EDTA for titration. What is the concentration in grams per liter of $Zn(NO_3)_2$ in the solution?
6. A 1.200 gm. sample of Calcium Stearate (N.F. XIV, 778) was treated with HCl to liberate the Ca^{++} which was then titrated with 0.0500 M EDTA solution, 40.0 ml. being required. What is the percent calcium expressed as CaO in the sample?
7. A solution of $MgCl_2$ (25.00 ml.) was treated with an excess (50.00 ml.) of 0.0220 M EDTA solution, and the excess EDTA was titrated with 20.70 ml. of 0.0250 M $ZnCl_2$. What was the concentration in grams per 100 ml. of the $MgCl_2$ solution?

ANSWERS

1. 40.3 percent
2. 29.2 mg.
3. 0.0786 gm.
4. 40.3 ml.
5. 119 gm./L.
6. 9.35 percent
7. 0.222 gm./100 ml.

Chapter 6

Oxidation-Reduction Equilibria

So far we have been concerned with a few simple equilibria in which the reaction, whether neutralization, precipitation, or complex formation, involved no change in the valence of the participating ions. We come now to a situation in which such a change is involved: reactions during the course of which electrons are gained or lost. Such reactions are called *oxidation-reduction (redox) reactions*. Oxidation is a *loss* of electrons; reduction is a *gain*. The *oxidizing agent* is that which does the oxidizing thereby becoming reduced, i.e., it gains electrons. The reverse is true for the *reducing agent*. As in acid-base reactions (p. 20), one cannot exist without the other; for everything oxidized, something must be reduced. As long as the reaction does not cause the removal of one form or the other, such reactions can also be described as equilibria in which

$$\text{oxidant}_1 + \text{reductant}_2 \leftrightharpoons \text{oxidant}_2 + \text{reductant}_1.$$

We can refer again to an experiment done in an earlier chemistry course in which zinc was dissolved in acid to produce hydrogen:

$$Zn^\circ + 2\,HCl \leftrightharpoons ZnCl_2 + H_2$$

The process takes place in two steps:

Eq. 1 $$Zn^\circ - 2e \leftrightharpoons Zn^{++}$$

Eq. 2 $$2\,H^+ + 2e \leftrightharpoons H_2$$

The zinc was oxidized to Zn^{++} (lost electrons); the hydrogen ions were reduced to hydrogen gas (gained electrons).

You may also remember putting a clean iron nail into a solution of copper sulfate and after a few minutes seeing a coating of bright copper plating out on the nail. This can be described by the following equations:

Eq. 3 $$Fe^\circ - 2e \leftrightharpoons Fe^{++}$$

Eq. 4 $$Cu^{++} + 2e \leftrightharpoons Cu^\circ$$

overall $$CuSO_4 + Fe^\circ \leftrightharpoons Cu^\circ + FeSO_4$$

Notice that we have divided this reaction into two half-reactions, one representing the oxidizing step, the other the reducing step. Notice too that a valence change is involved, as many electrons are lost as are gained. This makes writing a balanced equation for redox reactions somewhat more complicated than the simpler equations we worked with earlier. Not only must they be balanced with respect to the atoms involved, but they must be balanced electronically as well. There are a few simple rules by which this may be accomplished:

1. Know the reaction—the starting materials and the products—under study.
2. Write the half-reactions.
3. Balance each of these with respect to atoms, using H^+, H_2O, or OH^- depending on the conditions under which the reaction is run.
4. Balance each with respect to electrons gained and lost.
5. Write a balanced partial equation.
6. Add the incidental ions—those which take no part in the oxidation or the reduction—necessary to form the complete compounds in the fully balanced equation.

An example should make this process clear. The U.S.P. assay of hydrogen peroxide solution involves its oxidation to elemental oxygen by means of potassium permanganate in acid solution. Knowing this, we can write the half-reactions:

Eq. 5 $$H_2O_2 \leftrightarrows O_2 + 2\,H^+$$

Eq. 6 $$MnO_4^- + H^+ \leftrightarrows Mn^{++} + H_2O$$

Equation 5 is balanced with respect to atoms as it stands; we can balance Equation 6 by writing:

$$MnO_4^- + 8\,H^+ \leftrightarrows Mn^{++} + 4\,H_2O.$$

However, we do not yet have an electron balance; Equation 5 involves a loss of 2e (electrons) and Equation 6 a gain of 5e. We must therefore multiply Equation 5 by 5 and Equation 6 by 2 to equalize the gain and loss of electrons. This yields

Eq. 7 $$5 \times [H_2O_2 - 2e \leftrightarrows O_2 + 2\,H^+]$$

Eq. 8 $$2 \times [MnO_4^- + 8\,H^+ + 5e \leftrightarrows Mn^{++} + 4\,H_2O]$$

Eq. 9 overall $$5\,H_2O_2 + 2\,MnO_4^- + 16\,H^+ \leftrightarrows 5\,O_2 + 2\,Mn^{++} + 8\,H_2O + 10\,H^+$$

Notice that we can subtract 10 H^+ from each side of the equation to give

Eq. 10 $$5\,H_2O_2 + 2\,MnO_4^- + 6\,H^+ \leftrightarrows 5\,O_2 + 2\,Mn^{++} + 8\,H_2O.$$

Now put in the *incidental* or *spectator ions* and we have a complete, balanced equation which represents the reaction between hydrogen peroxide and potassium permanganate:

Eq. 11 $$5\,H_2O_2 + 2\,KMnO_4 + 3\,H_2SO_4 \leftrightarrows 5\,O_2 + 2\,MnSO_4 + K_2SO_4 + 8\,H_2O.$$

The easiest way to become familiar with these reactions is to study a few examples. Try to balance the equation which describes the solution of copper in nitric acid:

$$Cu^\circ + HNO_3 \leftrightarrows Cu(NO_3)_2 + NO + H_2O$$

Iodine and iodides figure prominently in redox reactions; they are so often used that the special term *iodometry* was coined to describe them. Most of these reactions involve double titrations in which the iodine liberated in one reaction is titrated by means of a second.

Example 1. Potassium dichromate oxidizes iodide to iodine in acid solution:

$$\begin{array}{l} Cr_2O_7^{=} + 14\,H^+ + 6e \leftrightharpoons 2\,Cr^{3+} + 7\,H_2O \\ 3 \times [2\,I^- - 2e \leftrightharpoons I_2] \\ \hline Cr_2O_7^{=} + 14\,H^+ + 6\,I^- \leftrightharpoons 2\,Cr^{3+} + 3\,I_2 + 7\,H_2O \end{array}$$

The liberated iodine is now titrated with sodium thiosulfate:

$$\begin{array}{l} I_2 + 2e \leftrightharpoons 2\,I^- \\ 2\,S_2O_3^{=} - 2e \leftrightharpoons S_4O_6^{=} \\ \hline I_2 + 2\,S_2O_3^{=} \leftrightharpoons 2\,I^- + S_4O_6^{=} \end{array}$$

From the second reaction we see that 2 mM. of $S_2O_3^{=}$ are required to react with 1 mM. of I_2, and from the first reaction that 6 mM. of I^- are required to react with 1 mM. of $K_2Cr_2O_7$. Hence

$$6\text{ mM. } S_2O_3^{=} = 1\text{ mM. } K_2Cr_2O_7$$

Example 2. Iodate reacts with iodide as follows:

$$IO_3^- + 5\,I^- + 6\,H^+ \leftrightharpoons 3\,I_2 + 3\,H_2O$$

This case is unusual in that both the oxidant and the reductant yield the same product. Divide the reaction into its half-reactions:

$$\begin{array}{l} 2\,IO_3^- + 12\,H^+ + 10e \leftrightharpoons I_2 + 6\,H_2O \\ 5 \times [2\,I^- - 2e \leftrightharpoons I_2] \\ \hline 2\,IO_3^- + 10\,I^- + 12\,H^+ \leftrightharpoons 6\,I_2 + 6\,H_2O \end{array}$$

The liberated iodine is titrated with thiosulfate exactly as in Example 1.

From the equations for the thiosulfate titration, it is clear that $2\,S_2O_3^{=} = I_2$, and from the equation for the iodate reaction that $6\,I_2 = 2\,IO_3^-$. It follows that $12\,S_2O_3^{=} = 2\,IO_3^-$ or that $S_2O_3^{=} = IO_3^-/6$. This titration is similar to one suggested as a laboratory experiment at the end of this chapter. In it Strong Iodine Solution U.S.P., sometimes called Lugol's solution, is assayed for its content of iodine (approximately 5 gm.) and potassium iodide (approximately 10 gm.).

Example 3. A standard solution of potassium arsenite (0.05 M = 0.1 N) is used to determine the iodine in a sample (e.g., 5.0 ml.) of Lugol's solution.

$$\begin{array}{l} AsO_2^- + 2\,H_2O - 2e \leftrightharpoons AsO_4^{\equiv} + 4\,H^+ \\ I_2 + 2e \leftrightharpoons 2\,I^- \\ \hline AsO_2^- + I_2 + 2\,H_2O \leftrightharpoons H_2AsO_4^- + 2\,HI \end{array}$$

Had we taken a sample of 20.0 ml. of arsenite solution,

$$20.0 \text{ ml.} \times 0.05\text{ M} = 1\text{ mM. } KAsO_2 = 1\text{ mM. } I_2 = 254\text{ mg./5 ml.} = 5.08\text{ gm./100 ml.}$$

Now the iodide formed by this reaction PLUS the iodide originally present in the Lugol's solution (i.e., total iodide) is determined by titration with standard (0.05 M) KIO_3.

$$\begin{array}{c} IO_3^- + 6\,H^+ + 4e \leftrightharpoons I^+ + 3\,H_2O \\ 2 \times [I^- - 2e \leftrightharpoons I^+] \\ \hline IO_3^- + 2\,I^- + 6\,H^+ \leftrightharpoons 3\,I^+ + 3\,H_2O \end{array}$$

For every millimole of KIO_3 used, we oxidized 2 mM. of KI. For a 50.0 ml. sample, 50.0 × 0.05 = 2.50 mM. which corresponds to 2 × 2.50 = 5.00 mM. total KI oxidized. But 2.00 mM. of this was formed from iodine in the first step, hence 5.00 − 2.00 = 3.00 mM. represents the KI originally present in 5.0 ml. of Lugol's solution.

$$3.00\text{ mM./5 ml.} = 60.0\text{ mM./100 ml.}$$

and $$60.0 \times 166\text{ (mol. wt. of KI)} = 9.96\text{ gm./100 ml.}$$

Example 4. An interesting application of a redox reaction is the "Breathalyzer" used by many police departments to determine driver drunkenness. A measured volume of expired air is bubbled through a standard acidic solution of potassium chromate; alcohol is thereby oxidized to acetic acid:

$$\begin{array}{l} 4 \times [CrO_4^= + 8\,H^+ + 3e \leftrightharpoons Cr^{3+} + 4\,H_2O] \\ 3 \times [C_2H_6O + H_2O - 4e \leftrightharpoons C_2H_4O_2 + 4\,H^+] \\ \hline 4\,CrO_4^= + 3\,C_2H_6O + 32\,H^+ \leftrightharpoons 4\,Cr^{3+} + 3\,C_2H_4O_2 + 12\,H^+ + 13\,H_2O \end{array}$$

Note that 12 H^+ and 3 H_2O can be subtracted from each side of the equation. The decrease in intensity of the deep yellow color of the chromate ion is a measure of the amount of alcohol oxidized.

The problem of determining end-points in redox reactions is really no different than we have encountered in other cases. Potassium permanganate is deep violet in color and, when used in titrations, serves as its own indicator inasmuch as the manganous ion is colorless in dilute solution. The brown color of iodine is not as easily observed. However, we can take advantage of the deep blue color which it forms with starch and use this as an indicator, titrating either to the appearance or disappearance of this color as the situation demands. In addition, there exists a selection of oxidation-reduction indicators which have one color in the oxidized form and another in the reduced form. An indicator with an equivalence point close to the equivalence point of the reaction is chosen, as with the pH indicators studied earlier.

THINGS TO REMEMBER

OXIDATION: A loss of electrons
REDUCTION: A gain of electrons
OXIDIZING AGENTS become reduced
REDUCING AGENTS become oxidized

Experiment 6. Assay of Strong Iodine Solution (Lugol's Solution)

1. Prepare a 0.0500 M solution of potassium iodate by accurately weighing 2.6750 gm. of KIO_3 and dissolving it in approximately 100 ml. of distilled water in a beaker. Transfer the solution quantitatively to a 250 ml. volumetric flask, fill to mark with distilled water, and mix thoroughly.

2. A solution of 0.05 M potassium arsenite will be provided.

3. *Assay for Iodine*. Pipet 5.00 ml. of strong iodine solution into each of three 250 ml. glass-stoppered conical flasks, add about 10 ml. of water to one sample, and titrate with the standard arsenite solution. You may run the arsenite solution into the flask rather rapidly, with good shaking, at the beginning. When the brown color of the iodine solution becomes yellow, add 1 or 2 ml. of starch solution and complete the titration just to the disappearance of the blue color. Record the amount of arsenite used.

4. *Assay for Potassium Iodide*. To the titrated solution above, add 25 ml. of hydrochloric acid and cool the mixture by swirling the flask under the cold water tap or immersing it in ice for a few minutes. Add 5 ml. of chloroform. Add a few milliliters of the iodate solution from a buret, stopper the flask, and shake well. Unstopper the flask and wash the stopper with a squirt from your wash bottle making sure the wash liquid enters the titration flask. Continue the titration in this manner until the purple color begins to disappear from the chloroform layer. As the end-point nears, add the iodate dropwise, with vigorous shaking; the chloroform layer becomes clear, virtually colorless. Allow the mixture to stand for 5 min.; if color returns to the chloroform layer, titrate further. Record the amount of iodate used. Repeat the titration for the other two samples.

The principle behind this iodometric titration, an oxidation-reduction reaction, has been discussed in detail (p. 47); refer to this discussion for the methods used in the calculation of the quantity of the constituents of Strong Iodine Solution, and express your results in terms of grams per 100 ml. of iodine and potassium iodide.

Experiment 7. Assay of Hydrogen Peroxide Solutions

Standardization of $KMnO_4$. A solution of approximately 0.1 N (0.02 M) potassium permanganate will be provided. Accurately weigh three samples of primary standard sodium oxalate of approximately 125 mg. each and transfer these quantitatively to 400 ml. beakers using about 200 ml. of distilled water containing 10 ml. of 1:1 sulfuric acid. Heat the solution to boiling, making sure that all of the sodium oxalate has dissolved. Now titrate the hot solution with the permanganate solution taking care to add no more than about 10 ml./min. The solution should be stirred vigorously during the titration. The end-point will be recognized by the persistence of the purple color of the permanganate solution. Record the buret readings and calculate the normality of the $KMnO_4$ expressing the result as the mean of your three determinations.

Assay of Hydrogen Peroxide. Pipet 2.0 ml. of your unknown hydrogen peroxide solution into each of three 125 ml. Erlenmeyer flasks and add 20 ml. of distilled water to each. Add 20 ml. of dilute (10 percent w/v) sulfuric acid and titrate with $KMnO_4$ solution to a permanent light pink end-point.

Write and balance the equation for the reaction and calculate the percentage of your hydrogen peroxide solution as the average of the three determinations.

PROBLEMS

1. Balance the following equations and express equivalents of reducing agent in terms of oxidizing agent.

Example.

$$Sb_2O_3 + I_2 + H_2O \leftrightharpoons Sb_2O_5 + HI$$

$$Sb^{3+} \xrightarrow{-2e} Sb^{5+}$$

$$I_2 \xrightarrow{+2e} 2\,I^-$$

$$Sb^{3+} + I_2 \leftrightharpoons Sb^{5+} + 2\,I^-$$

$$Sb_2O_3 + 2\,I_2 + 2\,H_2O \leftrightharpoons Sb_2O_5 + 4\,HI \quad \text{and} \quad I_2/2 = Sb_2O_3/4$$

(a) $CdS + HCl + I_2 \leftrightharpoons CdCl_2 + HI + S$
(b) $Cl_2 + KI \leftrightharpoons KCl + I_2$
(c) $K_2Cr_2O_7 + KI + H_2SO_4 \leftrightharpoons K_2SO_4 + Cr_2(SO_4)_3 + I_2 + H_2O$
(d) $NaCNS + KMnO_4 + H_2SO_4 \leftrightharpoons K_2SO_4 + MnSO_4 + NaCN + H_2O$
(e) $FeCl_3 + KI \leftrightharpoons KCl + FeCl_2 + I_2$
(f) $MnO_2 + FeSO_4 + H_2SO_4 \leftrightharpoons MnSO_4 + Fe_2(SO_4)_3 + H_2O$
(g) $V_2O_5 + Zn + H_2SO_4 \leftrightharpoons ZnSO_4 + V_2O_2 + H_2O$
(h) $H_2S + I_2 \leftrightharpoons HI + S$
(i) $Ti_2(SO_4)_3 + Fe_2(SO_4)_3 \leftrightharpoons Ti(SO_4)_2 + FeSO_4$

2. Hypochlorite solutions, which are used as disinfectants and bleaches, oxidize iodide in acid solution according to:

$$OCl^- + 2\,I^- + 2\,H^+ \leftrightharpoons Cl^- + I_2 + H_2O$$

The iodine can then be determined by use of thiosulfate. Calculate the percent sodium hypochlorite in a solution which required 67.2 ml. of 0.100 N thiosulfate ($Na_2S_2O_3$) for titration. Assume that 100 ml. of OCl^- was added.

3. In the equation given in 1(d) above 1.000 ml. of 0.1000 N $KMnO_4$ is equivalent to how many milligrams of sodium thiocyanate?
4. 0.2800 gm. of pure copper metal was dissolved in acid. After appropriate adjustment of solution conditions, an excess of KI was added, and the liberated iodine was titrated with 0.1050 N sodium thiosulfate. How many milliliters of sodium thiosulfate were used?
5. An aqueous solution contains both sulfuric and oxalic acids. With adequate amounts of sample on hand, devise a procedure for the analysis of both substances in the mixture.
6. 0.3420 gm. of sodium oxalate was titrated with 0.1024 N $KMnO_4$ of which 40.15 ml. were used. How pure is the sodium oxalate?
7. A sample of 0.2015 gm. of pure arsenious oxide (As_2O_3) was used to standardize a potassium permanganate solution, 39.80 ml. were used in the titration. Calculate the normality of the $KMnO_4$. (*Hint:* As_2O_3 when dissolved in water gives H_3AsO_3, and it is this which is actually oxidized by the permanganate.
8. If you think you have the idea well in hand, try this one: A ceric sulfate solution was standardized by titration against a solution of 0.2005 gm. of As_2O_3 (mol. wt. = 197.84), a volume of 42.2 ml. being used. Potassium iodide was then used to treat 20.0 ml. of this ceric sulfate solution and the iodine thus liberated was titrated using 25.7 ml. of a

sodium thiosulfate solution. What volume of this thiosulfate solution would be required to titrate the iodine liberated by the treatment of 0.1000 gm. of KIO_3 (mol. wt. 214) with an excess of KI in acid solution?

ANSWERS

1. (a) $I_2 = CdS$
   (b) $KI = Cl_2/2$
   (c) $KI = K_2Cr_2O_7/6$
   (d) $KMnO_4/5 = NaCNS/6$
   (e) $KI = FeCl_3$
   (f) $MnO_2/2 = FeSO_4$
   (g) $Zn/2 = V_2O_5/6$
   (h) $H_2S/2 = I_2/2$
   (i) $Ti = Fe$
2. 0.25 percent
3. 1.350 mg.
4. 42.0 ml.
6. 80.6 percent
7. 0.1025 N
8. 37.5 ml.

Chapter 7

Potentiometry

We began our discussions of chemical equilibria with those based on the simple fact of the ionization of water and have built an approach to more complex equilibria which, nonetheless, lend themselves to the same kind of mathematical treatment. At this point, it seems appropriate to attempt to answer a few questions which have been lurking in the background. We have referred to the equilibrium constants K_a, K_b, K_{eq}, K_f, K_{sp}, and K_w. Where do these come from? How are they derived? And, however broad the selection of indicators for titrimetric analyses may be, what resources are available to us in the event solutions are too highly colored, too dark, or too turbid for proper visual estimation of the end-point?

It is easiest to approach this matter by means of the redox reactions we have just studied. Such reactions involve the transfer of electrons from one substance to another:

$$S_1 - 3e \rightleftharpoons S_1^{3+} \quad (1)$$

$$S_2^{3+} + 3e \rightleftharpoons S_2 \quad (2)$$

Instead of having these reactions take place simultaneously in a beaker or flask, let us imagine them separated but connected by a wire including a switch (see figure below). When the switch is closed, the electrons generated by the reaction (1) flow through the wire and are used in the reaction (2). Electrons in motion we define as electricity or electromotive force (EMF). If we measure this flow of electricity, we have a measure of the overall reaction. As long as the current flows, we know that the reaction is in progress; when all of S_1 is used up, it is over. This reaction is called an electrochemical cell; oxidation takes place at the *anode,* reduction at the *cathode.* If the electron flow is spontaneous, we have a galvanic cell, i.e., a battery. If voltage must be applied to make the reaction take

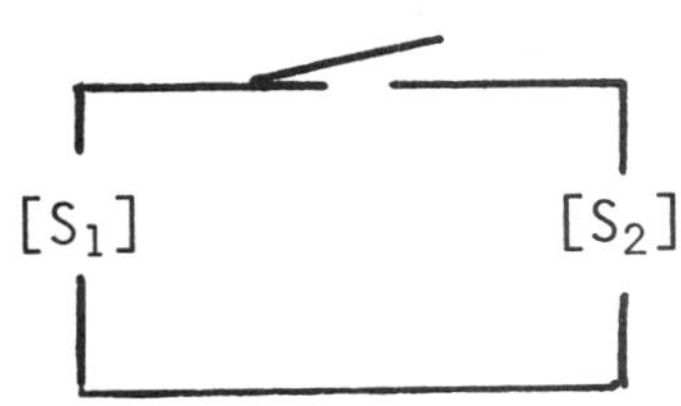

place, we have an electrolytic cell of which the familiar process of plating on metals is an example. While this latter type of cell does have analytical application, we will concern ourselves with the former.

There are problems in measuring the voltages of galvanic cells. Consider a simple one like this:

$$Zn^{\circ} / Zn^{++}\ 1\ M\ //\ Cu^{++}\ 1\ M / Cu^{\circ}$$

Two half-cells are represented, two half-reactions which, on the basis of our recent experience, we may write as:

$$\text{(anode)} \qquad Zn^{\circ} - 2e \leftrightarrow Zn^{++}\ \text{(oxidation)}$$

$$\text{(cathode)} \qquad Cu^{++} + 2e \leftrightarrow Cu^{\circ}\ \text{(reduction)}$$

These reactions take place as soon as contact is made between the copper and zinc plates, and a given EMF is produced. This EMF will change for two reasons: (1) the concentration of Zn^{++} will increase in that half of the cell while the concentration of Cu^{++} will decrease because of plating out of the copper and the initial voltage will eventually drop (transistor batteries do wear out), and (2) the voltage of the cell as a whole is influenced primarily by the concentration of the ions near the surfaces of the electrodes and not so greatly by those in solution farther away. These influences are difficult to measure because they keep changing.

What we would like to do is measure the voltage of the cell without these changes taking place. This can be done by introducing a known variable voltage to oppose that of the Zn/Cu cell. When no current flows (null point), voltages are equal and opposite, hence the known applied voltage becomes a measure of the voltage of the cell.

Perhaps this is as good a point as any to introduce the conventions and simple explanations concerning electrochemical cells which will aid in the understanding of what follows. We write equations describing these cells so that the half-cell at which oxidation occurs is at the left (half-reaction$_1$). The half-cell on the left thus becomes the anode (oxidation) and negatively charged because it is here that electrons are discharged. Reduction takes place in the half-cell written at the right (half-reaction$_2$) which is the cathode. The total voltage developed by the cell is the sum of $E_1 + E_2$. *There is no relationship between the sign of E and the signs of the electrodes.* The sign of E is a thermodynamic concept; if it is (+) the reaction occurs spontaneously; if (−) it is nonspontaneous. The sign of the electrode is an electrochemical concept and is invariant; oxidation occurs at the anode, reduction at the cathode. Further, as we mentioned earlier, the actual potentiometric measurement involves no real current flow (use of a null-point instrument) so what we are really measuring is a *tendency* for a reaction to take place which might be realized only when the terminals are connected and the cell allowed to operate.

Now let's return to our Zn/Cu cell, the voltage of which we were able to measure by the null-point technique. While this gives us a measure of the cell voltage for the overall reaction, what we would really like to have is a method to measure the voltage of an individual half-cell reaction. It is impossible to give this an absolute value for, as we have learned, there can be no oxidation without simultaneous reduction. It becomes necessary to measure what we want relative to some arbitrarily chosen standard.

This standard is the half-cell composed of the normal hydrogen electrode (NHE or SHE). It consists of a specially prepared platinum electrode in a solution of 1 M in H^+ over which is bubbled hydrogen gas at 1 atm. pressure at 25°C. The half-reaction

$$H_2 - 2e \rightleftharpoons 2\,H^+$$

is assigned an arbitrary voltage, E°, of 0.0000 v. We can now measure the E of any other half-cell by measuring the voltage of a galvanic cell in which SHE is the other half. For example,

$$\text{Pt, } H_2 \,/\, 1\text{ M HCl} \,//\, \text{AgCl} \,/\, \text{Ag}^\circ$$

for which the half-reactions are:

$$H_2 - 2e \rightleftharpoons 2\,H^+$$

$$2\,\text{AgCl} + 2e \rightleftharpoons 2\,\text{Ag}^\circ + 2\,\text{Cl}^-$$

and $$H_2 + 2\,\text{AgCl} \rightleftharpoons 2\,H^+ + 2\,\text{Cl}^- + 2\,\text{Ag}^\circ.$$

If now we measure the voltage of this cell, we record a value of 0.2222 v. A positive voltage indicates that, were the terminals connected, current would flow and the reaction would be spontaneous. As indicated previously, the hydrogen electrode is the anode, the Ag/AgCl electrode is the cathode.

The Zn/Zn^{++} half-cell can be set up vs. the SHE in the same way:

$$\text{Zn}^\circ/\text{Zn}^{++}\ 1\text{ M} \,//\, H^+\ 1\text{ M} \,/\, H_2\text{, Pt}$$

The half reactions:

$$\text{Zn}^\circ - 2e \rightleftharpoons \text{Zn}^{++} \text{ (oxidation)}$$

$$2\,H^+ + 2e \rightleftharpoons H_2 \text{ (reduction)}$$

$$\text{Zn}^\circ + 2\,H^+ \rightleftharpoons \text{Zn}^{++} + H_2$$

Zinc is being oxidized hence this is the anode; H^+ is being reduced at the cathode. Zinc furnished the electrons, hence this terminal is – vs. the SHE. Measurement of the voltage gives a value of +0.76 v., therefore the reaction is spontaneous as written. This is how it happens that you can produce hydrogen by dissolving zinc in acid—the experiment to which we referred earlier. We can do the same for any other half-cell reaction and create tables relating one redox reaction to another; those which are + relative to SHE are spontaneous and will take place as written. A table for some common redox reactions is given in the Appendix.

We will now make some analytical applications of these concepts. Without going into the thermodynamic, electrochemical, and mathematical theory necessary to demonstrate the fact, we will accept here that it can be shown for any half-cell that

$$E = E^\circ - 0.059/n \cdot \log Q \text{ (sometimes L)}$$

where E = observed potential, E° = standard potential vs. SHE, n = number of electrons transferred in the redox reaction, and Q = activity quotient. This expression is called the *Nernst equation*. You will recall that in our use of equilibrium constants we used concentration in place of activity,

so that $$aA + bB \rightleftharpoons mM + nN$$

and $[M]^m\,[N]^n/[A]^a\,[B]^b = K_{eq}$ instead of Q,

realizing that this held *for dilute solutions only;* that K is not constant for high concentrations. To cover all cases, we should be using the term *activity* wherein the activity of a given solute may depend on its own concentration as well as on the concentration of other solutes in the solution. With this in mind, we will continue to use "concentration" rather than "activity" understanding that we are dealing with dilute solutions when we do so.

Perhaps the best way to understand how these principles apply to analytical problems is through a few examples. We have defined the SHE as Pt, H_2, 1 M in H^+ at 1 atm. and 25°C. with E = 0.0000 v. Suppose we were to measure it against another hydrogen half-cell with pure water in place of 1 M H^+. By definition, $[H^+]$ in pure water is 10^{-7} M. Applying the Nernst equation,

$$E = E^\circ - \frac{0.059}{2} \log [aH^+]^2/[aH_2]$$

We can use $[H^+]$ instead of $[aH^+]$ because 10^{-7} is a very dilute solution of H^+; the activity of H_2 at 1 atm. and 25°C = 1; therefore:

$$\begin{aligned} E &= 0.0000 - 0.0295 \log [10^{-7}]^2 \\ &= +0.413. \end{aligned}$$

Now let's turn the problem around. An aqueous solution measured against the SHE showed a potential of 0.413 v. What is its pH?

$$\begin{aligned} E &= E^\circ - 0.059/2 \log [H^+]^2 \\ 0.413 &= 0.00 - 0.0295 \log [H^+]^2 \\ \log [H^+]^2 &= -0.413/0.0295 = -14 \\ \log [H^+] &= -7.0 \quad \text{and} \quad pH = 7.0 \end{aligned}$$

This is a method for measuring the pH of aqueous solutions which we will discuss in more detail later.

Proceeding a step further, let us apply the Nernst equation to our Zn/Cu cell for which the overall reaction may be written:

$$Zn^\circ + Cu^{++} \leftrightharpoons Zn^{++} + Cu^\circ$$

By the conventions we have adopted,

$$E_{cell} = E_2^\circ + E_1^\circ - 0.059/n \log \frac{[aZn^{++}]\,[aCu^\circ]}{[aZn^\circ]\,[aCu^{++}]}.$$

By definition the activity of a solid is 1, and since the cell was set up with the activities of Zn^{++} and Cu^{++} equal, we have

$$\begin{aligned} E_{cell} &= E_1^\circ + E_2^\circ - 0.059/2 \log Q \\ &= 0.76 + 0.34 = 1.10 \text{ v.} \end{aligned}$$

Generally, then,

$$E_{cell} = E^{\circ}_{right} + E^{\circ}_{left} - 0.059/n \log Q$$

in which Q = activity product of cell *product ions* divided by activity product of cell *reactant ions*. These calculations can be used to determine a number of things of concern to the analytical chemist.

1. *Equilibrium Constant*. The reaction representing the oxidation of Sn^{++} by Fe^{3+} can be divided into half-reactions as follows:

$$Sn^{2+} - 2e \leftrightarrow Sn^{4+}$$

$$2\,Fe^{3+} + 2e \leftrightarrow 2\,Fe^{2+}$$

As a cell

$$E = E^{\circ}_1 + E^{\circ}_2 \frac{-0.059}{2} \log \frac{[Fe^{2+}]^2\,[Sn^{4+}]}{[Fe^{3+}]^2\,[Sn^{2+}]}$$

At equilibrium

$$E = 0 = -0.15 + 0.77 - 0.0295 \log K_{eq}$$

$$\log K_{eq} = 0.62/0.0295 = 21 \quad \text{and} \quad K_{eq} = 10^{21}$$

2. *Solubility Product*. Consider the reaction between Ag^+ and Cl^- to form AgCl. This can be divided into half-reactions as follows:

$$Ag^{\circ} - e \leftrightarrow Ag^+$$

$$AgCl + e \leftrightarrow Ag^{\circ} + Cl^-$$

As a cell, $E = E^{\circ}_1 + E^{\circ}_2 - 0.059 \log [Ag^+]\,[Cl^-]$, and at equilibrium

$$0 = -0.799 + 0.22 - 0.059 \log K_{sp}$$

$$\log K_{sp} = -0.579/0.059 = -9.81$$

$$K_{sp} = 1.55 \times 10^{-10}$$

3. *Determination of pH*. Previously we saw that a nonstandard hydrogen electrode, using pure water instead of 1 M H^+, showed a potential difference when measured against the SHE, thereby reflecting changes in pH. The use of hydrogen electrodes entails many problems. They are elegant but "touchy" pieces of equipment, not particularly easy to set up, difficult to maintain, easily poisoned, and they require hydrogen gas. We might improve matters somewhat by removing at least one of them in the experiment which was described earlier by using some other electrode as a reference in place of the SHE. Suppose we have

$$\text{Ref. electrode} // H^+/ H_2, Pt$$

where $[H^+]$ is unknown. Applying the Nernst equation

$$E_{cell} = E^{\circ}_{ref} - 0.059/n \log [H^+]^2$$

$$E_{cell} - E^{\circ}_{ref} - 0.059/2 \log [H^+]^2$$

$$\text{or} \quad E_{cell} - E^{\circ}_{ref} = 0.059 \text{ pH}$$

If E°_{ref} is determined against the SHE independently, E_{cell} becomes a measure of the pH. A reference electrode commonly used for this purpose is the saturated calomel electrode (SCE). This is composed of calomel, solid Hg_2Cl_2, in saturated KCl:

$$Hg_2Cl_2 + 2e \leftrightarrows 2\,Hg^{\circ} + 2\,Cl^-$$

Since the potential depends only on the activity of the Cl^-, it is not influenced by H^+ and can be used *vs*. SHE for the determination of this ion; E = 0.2415 v.

We can now eliminate the SHE entirely by using what is known as the glass electrode. This is actually a silver/silver chloride electrode separated from the solution to be measured by a thin glass membrane which, by reason of its special formulation, is sensitive to H^+ through ion exchange phenomena rather than electron transfer. It looks, and is, rather complex:

$$\underset{E_1}{Hg^{\circ}/Hg_2Cl_2},\ \underset{E_2}{HCl/}\ \text{sample solution}\ \underset{E_3}{//}\ \underset{E_4}{AgCl, HCl}\ \underset{E_5}{/\ Ag^{\circ}}$$

where E_1 = E for the SCE,
E_2 = liquid junction potential between the solution and the SCE,
E_3 = boundary potential between the glass membrane and the solution,
E_4 = boundary potential between the glass membrane and HCl, and
E_5 = E for the Ag/AgCl electrode.

E_{cell} is the sum of all these potentials developed in the cell when in use. It is equal to 0.059 pH + a constant (k) which accounts for all of the contributing potentials except E_3 which cannot be determined precisely. The constant k is therefore determined for a given electrode by calibration using a buffer of known pH in the range of the pH to be anticipated in the determination. Thus, after "zeroing" the instrument, the pH meter becomes simply a voltmeter with the dial calibrated to read pH directly since pH = E_{cell} divided by 0.059.

4. *Acid-base Titrations*. It follows that an acid-base titration can be carried out using the pH meter as an indicator, a large change in voltage being observed at the equivalence point rather than a change of color of an indicator. A titration of hydrochloric acid using sodium hydroxide might be described by plotting the voltage, i.e., pH, recorded after each addition of base vs. the milliliters of sodium hydroxide used. The equivalence point is read at that volume of NaOH represented by the midpoint of the rapidly rising, straight line portion of the voltage curve (see figure p. 59).

5. *Precipitation Reactions*. We have already alluded to these reactions under our discussion of solubility product and its estimation. The indicator electrodes are usually made of the metal involved in the precipitate, e.g., Ag, Pb, Fe, etc.

6. *Oxidation-Reduction Reactions*. The indicator electrodes are made of a noble metal, e.g., gold or platinum, unaffected by redox reactions. The two half-reactions of the redox system are considered together as one half of the cell and the reference electrode as the other half. The SCE is often used as a reference electrode.

7. *Redox Indicators*. Obviously, if a redox titration is done potentiometrically, there is no need for an indicator to determine the equivalence point. However, to determine the

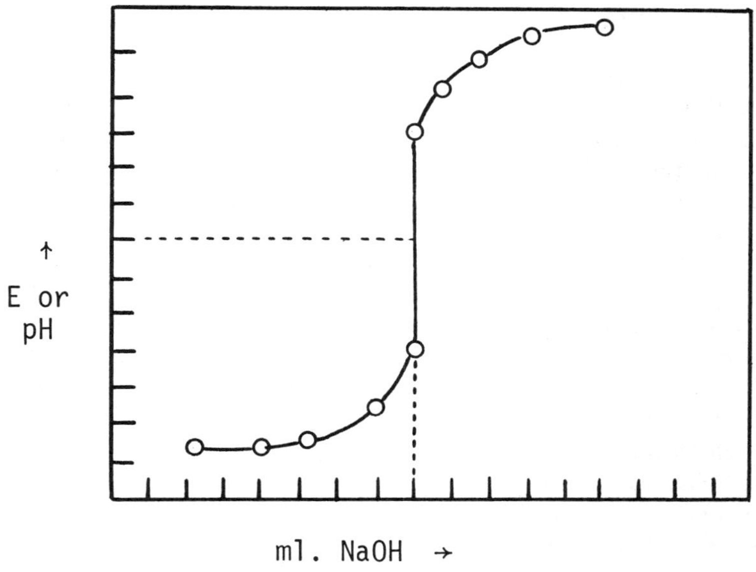

suitability of a particular redox indicator for a particular redox reaction, indicators can be treated like any other substance in a redox reaction:

$$E = E^0 - 0.059/n \log \text{reduced form} / \text{oxidized form}.$$

As we learned earlier, the sensitivity of the human eye is such that the ratio of one color to the other must be at least 10/1 in order to be seen clearly as a distinct change. Therefore:

$$E = E^0 - 0.059/n \log 10$$
$$= E^0 - 0.059/n.$$

As in other cases, E^0 v.s. SHE is used in such calculations, and E can be determined for the range over which an indicator will be useful in non-potentiometric titrations.

It should be mentioned that many indicators have color changes which are pH dependent as well as dependent on their oxidation state. Since many redox reactions are carried out in acid solution and since the amount of indicator usually added to a solution before titration is small, we have neglected this effect in our general discussion. While it is convenient to think of the change of an indicator as an equilibrium between its oxidized and reduced forms, not all useful indicators behave in this way. Some, such as diphenylamine and diphenylbenzidine, may be destructively oxidized by an excess of reagents, such as Ce^{4+} or $Cr_2O_7^{=}$, and cannot be reconverted to their reduced forms. Metal complexes are often used as redox indicators; a common example is ferrous phenanthroline (Ferroin) used in titrations involving iron and cerium salts. Some are highly fluorescent and are used in titrations in which the solutions themselves are too highly colored for easy visualization using traditional color-change indicators.

8. *Ion-Selective Electrodes.* A number of electrodes have become available in which the membrane potential is selective toward an ion or ions other than H^+. These may be glass membrane, precipitate impregnated, solid state, or liquid membrane electrodes depending on the application. Those using the principle of the glass membrane are similar in

construction to the pH glass electrode discussed above. The composition of the glass is modified so that it shows a higher affinity for a particular cation than it does for protons, so that membrane potential is primarily dependent on the concentration of the cation. Nonetheless, this type of electrode is still sensitive to the proton concentration of the solution, and to minimize interference by H^+ they are often used with solutions of high pH.

Precipitate impregnated electrodes normally consist of a membrane impregnated with an insoluble salt such as $BaSO_4$ which would, for example, function as a sulfate electrode. Electrodes sensitive to iodide, bromide, and chloride are readily prepared, as are those sensitive to phosphate, sulfate, and hydroxide ions. In electrodes of this type, lack of sensitivity and selectivity may limit their use. Their sensitivity is limited by the solubility of the salt contained in the membrane. Normally, they are sensitive to solution anion concentrations of about ten times the molar solubility of the precipitate. Using a $BaSO_4$ membrane as an example, its molar solubility of 10^{-5} limits the sensitivity of the electrode to $SO_4^=$ concentrations in the range of 10^{-4} M.

Solid state electrodes have a "membrane" made of a single crystal of a salt containing the ion of interest. The fluoride electrode, for example, consists of a crystal of lanthanum fluoride containing some europium to reduce electrical resistance. The selectivity of this electrode for fluoride vs. hydroxide is poor, and for this reason it is recommended that measurements be made at $pH < 8$.

An example of the liquid membrane electrode is the Ca-selective electrode which contains a liquid ion exchanger immiscible with water. This is held in place at the tip of the device by a porous membrane which facilitates contact between the solution and the membrane but minimizes mixing. The body of the electrode is filled with a solution of Ca^{++}.

For many determinations, these ion-selective electrodes have replaced the more classical methods for the assay of particular ions. For example, the fluoride electrode has been used to determine the concentration of F^- in products ranging from multivitamin preparations to gels used in the prevention of dental caries.

THINGS TO REMEMBER

$$E = E^\circ - \frac{0.059}{n} \log Q$$

$$E_{cell} = E^\circ_{oxid} + E^\circ_{red} - \frac{0.059}{n} \log Q$$

$$E = 0.059\, pH$$

Experiment 8. Potentiometric Assay of Nicotinic Acid

NOTES. A. The electrodes used in this experiment are delicate and expensive. Caution should be used in all operations involving them. At the conclusion of the experiment, make sure that they are left immersed in a beaker containing distilled water.

B. Prepare 0.1 N NaOH transferring by pipet 25.0 ml. of your standard 1.0 N solution into a 250 ml. volumetric flask and making up to volume. Make sure your pipet is "to deliver" and do not blow out the drops remaining in the tip after drainage.

1. A buffer solution with a pH of 7.0 will be supplied for standardization of your pH

meter. Take a small portion of it in a small beaker. Be sure the instrument is on "standby." Remove the beaker of distilled water from the electrode. Insert the electrode in the buffer solution carefully so that the tip is completely immersed. Depress the "read" button of your instrument, and note the pH after the instrument stabilizes. If it does not read exactly 7.0, adjust it so that it does. Again put the meter on "standby." Repeat the standardization. Wash off the electrode with distilled water from your wash bottle.

2. Set up the necessary apparatus as follows. To a tall-form 150 ml. beaker add 25.0 ml. (by pipet) of the nicotinic acid solution. Dilute it with an equal volume of water (from graduated cylinder). Place a magnetic stirring bar in the beaker and place the beaker on the magnetic stirrer. Carefully place the electrode at one side of the beaker so that the tip is covered by the solution but does not impede the movement of the stirring bar. Now set up a buret previously filled with 0.1 N NaOH so that the tip will deliver the titrant into the beaker. Carefully turn on the magnetic stirrer so that the bar rotates gently at the bottom of the beaker. When the solution is well mixed, read the pH and record this value.

3. Add 3 ml. of the titrant from the buret. Read the pH. Repeat the addition in 3 ml. increments until the pH of the solution reaches 11 to 12. Record both the amount of NaOH added and the pH of the resulting solution after each addition. Return the meter to "standby."

Examine your data and note the increments between which there was the greatest change in pH value. This range includes the equivalence point. Discard the sample, wash off the electrode with distilled water, and start over.

Repeat the third step, this time adding 0.5 ml. increments (see note below) of base from about 3 ml. before the equivalence point (as determined above) and 3 ml. after it, recording the amount added and the pH change as before. Return the meter to "standby," wash off the electrode and return it to the beaker of distilled water.

Using graph paper, plot milliliters of NaOH along the abcissa and the corresponding pH value along the ordinate. The end-point of the titration is determined by drawing a vertical line from the midpoint of the steepest part of the curve to the x-axis.

Calculate the amount of nicotinic acid in your sample and express the result as in grams per 100 ml.

> NOTE. Just before, and immediately after the equivalence point, add the titrant dropwise.

Experiment 9. Determination of Fluoride Concentration Using a Fluoride Electrode

This experiment is adapted from a procedure described by Jones, Heveran, and Senkowski.*

Standard Fluoride Stock Solution. Weigh exactly 221.0 mg. of sodium fluoride previously dried for 24 hr. at 100°C. Transfer it quantitatively to a 100 ml. volumetric flask and dissolve it in approximately 25 ml. of deionized water. Add 1 ml. of 0.1 N NaOH and dilute to volume with deionized water. Pipet 10.0 ml. of this solution into a second 100 ml. volumetric flask and dilute to volume with deionized water. The fluoride content of this solution is 0.1 mg./ml.

Tris Buffer Solution (TBS). This solution should be prepared the day it is to be used. Using a graduated cylinder add 500 ml. of 1.0 M tris (hydroxymethyl) aminomethane, primary

*Jones, B. C., Heveran, J. E., and Senkowski, B. Z.: *Specific ion electrode determination of fluoride in multivitamin preparations*. J. Pharm. Sci. 58:607, 1969.

standard grade, and 403 ml. of 1.0 M HCl to a 1 L. volumetric flask and dilute to final volume with deionized water. The pH of this solution is 7.5 ± 0.1.

Fluoride Standards. Students may work in groups of four. To a series of 100 ml. volumetric flasks, transfer by pipet 0.1, 0.25, 0.50, 1.2, and 5.0 ml. samples of the standard fluoride stock solution and dilute to volume with freshly prepared tris buffer solution (TBS). These solutions contain 0.01, 0.025, 0.05, 0.10, 0.20, and 0.50 mg./100 ml. fluoride.

Unknown Solution. Accurately weigh 20 Sodium Fluoride Tablets (U.S.P. XIX, 460) and determine the average weight per tablet. In a small mortar and pestle grind two tablets to a fine powder. Accurately weigh a portion equal to half a tablet. Transfer this material quantitatively to a 100 ml. volumetric flask and add 75 ml. of TBS. Heat on a steam bath for 20 to 30 min. and, after cooling to room temperature, make up to volume with TBS. Transfer approximately 35 ml. of the final solution to a glass-stoppered centrifuge tube and centrifuge for 10 min. Pipet 20.0 ml. of the clear centrifuged sample to a 100 ml. volumetric flask and dilute to volume with TBS.

Measurements. Transfer a portion of the solution to be measured to a 150 ml. beaker containing a Teflon-coated stirring bar and place the beaker on the magnetic stirrer. Carefully immerse the fluoride-selective electrode and measure the potential (millivolts) after stirring for 1 to 2 min. Do this for each of the standard solutions as well as for the unknown, carefully washing the electrode with deionized water between each use.

Calculations. Plot fluoride concentration (mg./100 ml.) against the potential (mV.) for each of the standards using semilog paper (1 cycle × 70 divisions). The fluoride concentration of the unknown solution is determined directly from this graph. To calculate the fluoride concentration of the original tablets, use the following proportion:

$$\frac{\text{Tablet F}^- \text{ concentration}}{\text{Average tablet weight}} = \frac{5 \times \text{F}^- \text{ concentration (from graph)}}{\text{Sample weight}}$$

PROBLEMS

1. Consider the following reaction:

$$Pb^\circ + 2\,Ag^+ + SO_4^= \leftrightharpoons PbSO_4 + 2\,Ag^\circ$$

   (a) Write the two half-reactions.
   (b) Write the expression for the EMF of the overall reaction.
   (c) If $[SO_4^=]$ is 0.5 M and $[Ag^+]$ is 0.003 M, calculate:
      (1) the EMF for the Pb, $PbSO_4$ half-reaction
      (2) the EMF for the Ag^+, Ag half-reaction
      (3) the EMF for the overall reaction given that

$$E^\circ \text{ for Pb, } PbSO_4 = 0.356\text{ v. and } E^\circ \text{ for } Ag^+\text{, Ag} = 0.800\text{ v.}$$

2. Balance the equation $H_2S + I_2 \leftrightharpoons HI + S$

   Calculate the equilibrium constant for this reaction given that E° for $S^=$, S° = −0.141v. and E° for I_2, I^- = 0.620 v.

3. Using pure water and the SHE show that E = 0.059pH.
4. Calculate the solubility product of silver iodide given that E° for AgI, Ag = 0.15 v. and E° for Ag, Ag^+ = −0.80 v.
5. Phenobarbital ($C_{12}H_{12}N_2O_3$, mol. wt. = 232.26) is determined potentiometrically (U.S.P. XIX,372) in aqueous solution (containing alcohol) by titration with 0.1 N NaOH. A sample of 0.4644g./100 ml. required 20.00 ml. of the base for titration. What was the EMF reading at the equivalence point? pK_a for phenobarbital = 7.29.
6. A saturated calomel electrode (SCE) was set up against a hydrogen electrode containing a 0.01 M solution of a weak acid. The voltage measured was 0.481. Calculate K_a for the acid.
7. A common method for the determination of iron involves its titration with ceric sulfate in which $Fe^{++} - e \rightarrow Fe^{3+}$ and $Ce^{4+} + e \rightarrow Ce^{3+}$. Calculate K_{eq} for the reaction if E° for the Fe^{++} reaction = −0.771 v. and E° for the Ce^{4+} reaction = 1.70 v.

ANSWERS

1. (c) (1) 0.347 v.
   (2) 0.651 v.
   (3) 0.998 v.
2. 2.51×10^{16}
4. 7.94×10^{-17}
5. 0.576 v.
6. 7.23×10^{-7}
7. 5.65×10^{15}

Chapter 8

Solvent Extraction

Many analytical problems involve mixtures from which it is necessary to isolate one or more of the ingredients for quantitative estimation. Familiar examples include the isolation of drugs from dosage forms (e.g., aspirin from tablets), drugs and their metabolites from body fluids (e.g., blood or urine), and medicinal constituents of plants (e.g., atropine from *Atropa belladonna*). Solvent extraction is a method widely used for this purpose.

Consider as an example a very simple case: a mixture of aspirin and lactose. One substance might be separated from the other by solution in a single solvent; aspirin is soluble in ether, lactose is not. Usually the matter is not as simple as this, and we are forced to take advantage of the differential solubility of a substance in a mixture of two (sometimes more) immiscible solvents. A mixture such as aspirin and lactose might be shaken with a mixture of ether and water. After equilibrium, the two layers could be separated and each evaporated to dryness. It would then be seen that most of the aspirin had been extracted into the ether while most of the lactose remained in the water. This process is called *liquid-liquid extraction*.

Such methods are based on the *Nernst distribution law* which simply states that the ratio of the concentration in one phase to that in the other is constant at constant temperature. As with other cases we have discussed, we are speaking strictly of activity, but for the usual practical applications, concentration may be used and we can express the relationship by means of a very simple equation in which

$$C_1/C_2 = K_d$$

C_1 being the concentration of solute in the lipid phase, C_2 the concentration in the aqueous phase, and K_d the distribution (or partition) coefficient. A simple approximation of K_d for a given substance and solvent combination may be made in a manner analogous to that just described. A quantity of substance not exceeding the weight soluble in either of the solvents is partitioned by thorough shaking with equal volumes of solvents in a separatory funnel. After equilibrium, the solvent layers are separated, evaporated to dryness, and the residues weighed. Calculation of K_d is done simply by determination of the ratio of the weights as described above.

A second method involves repetition of the experiment described above using several different sample weights of the substance. If, then, the concentrations of the substance in the lipid phases are plotted against the concentrations in the water phases, a graph is obtained (the partition isotherm) the slope of which is equal to K_d (see figure below). Note that K_d is not a function of the volume of the solvents used in the extraction nor will it be the same value for all solvent systems; the concentration in each phase will depend on the solubility of the substance in that phase. However, as we shall see, this is not to say that volume plays no part at all in the completeness of extraction nor that we are limited to a single extraction in order to achieve a quantitative separation.

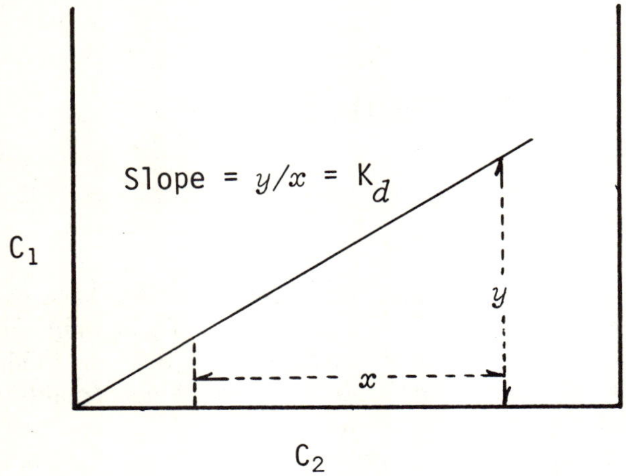

Let us examine this matter in more detail. It should be clear that unless K_d is large, a single extraction will give very poor quantitative separation. Assume aspirin to have K_d = 4.0 in an ether-blood serum (water) system. Suppose we were to extract a 15 ml. sample of blood serum with 15 ml. of ether. Since K = 4/1, it follows that only 80 percent of the aspirin will be extracted into the ether layer. The question now arises: Shall we use a larger amount of ether for the extraction or shall we extract several times—and if more than one time, how many times must we extract with small portions of ether in order to obtain a quantitative recovery?

If $K = C_1/C_2$, and we let V_1 = the volume of the lipid phase, V_2 the volume of the water phase, and p = the fraction in V_1 at equilibrium, then $(1 - p) = q$ = the fraction in V_2 at equilibrium. Therefore

$$K = \frac{[p/V_1]}{[(1 - p)/V_2]}$$

This can be solved for p as follows:

$$K = p/V_1 \times V_2/(1 - p) = V_2p/(V_1 - V_1p)$$

$$KV_1 - KV_1p = V_2p$$

$$\text{or} \quad KV_1 = V_2p + KV_1p = p(V_2 + KV_1)$$

$$\text{and} \quad KV_1/(V_2 + KV_1) = [KV_1/V_2]/[1 + KV_1/V_2] = p.$$

Let $V_1/V_2 = U$; then $p = KU/(KU + 1)$ and because $q = 1 - p$,

$$q = 1 - (KU/KU + 1) = 1/(KU + 1).$$

Let us apply this to the problem at hand: the extraction of aspirin from 15 ml. of serum. There are three things we might do:

1. *Single Extraction Using Equal Volumes of Solvents ($V_1 = V_2 = 15$ ml.).*

$$p = (4 \times 15)/15 + (4 \times 15) = 60/75 = 0.80$$

$$\text{or} \quad U = 15/15 = 1 \quad \text{and} \quad p = 4/(4 + 1) = 4/5 = 0.80$$

That is to say, 80 percent of the aspirin would be extracted by this procedure.

2. *Single Extraction Using Different Volumes of Solvents ($V_1 = 25$ ml., $V_2 = 15$ ml.).* In this case,

$$p = 4 \times 25/[15 + (4 \times 25)] = 100/115 = 0.87$$

$$\text{or} \quad U = 25/15 = 5/3 \quad \text{and} \quad p = 4(5/3)/[4(5/3) + 1] = (20/3)/(23/3) = 0.87$$

This is obviously more efficient but scarcely sufficiently so to be considered quantitative.

3. *Multiple Extraction.* Suppose we use 25 ml. of ether in five portions of 5 ml. each? As indicated above, for the first extraction:

$$p = 4 \times 5/[15 + (4 \times 5)] = 20/35 = 0.572$$

Extract No.		p *amount extracted (percent)*	q *amount remaining (percent)*
1		57.2	42.8
2	42.8 × 0.572	24.4	18.4
3	18.4 × 0.572	10.5	7.9
4	7.9 × 0.572	4.5	3.4
5	3.4 × 0.572	1.9	1.5
		98.5	

The total amount extracted in this way amounts to 98.5 percent of the aspirin present, an obvious improvement over the other methods.

In the first example above it was shown that 80 percent of the aspirin was recovered in a single extraction using equal volumes. If, as we have indicated, q is the amount remaining, it can be shown that for any number of extractions (n) the amount in the lipid phase of the nth extraction is pq^{n-1} and the amount remaining in the water phase after the nth extraction is q^n.

The problem might then be posed in the following way: for a substance having $K = 4$ in an ether-water system, how many extractions would be required to remove the solute quantitatively (99.99 percent recovery), assuming equal volumes of the two phases in a multiple extraction procedure? If $K = 4$, 80 percent is extracted (20 percent remains) after each extraction. We wish no more than 0.01 percent to remain after the final extraction, hence:

$$0.2^n = 0.0001$$

$$n \log 0.2 = \log 1 \times 10^{-4}$$

$$n(9.301 - 10) = -4.0$$

$$-0.699n = -4.0$$

$$n = -4.0/0.699 = 5.7$$

or, in round numbers, 6 times.

As you know, most of the compounds encountered in pharmaceutical analysis are either weak acids or bases. Their solubility will depend, therefore, on the pH of the system: the nonionized form of the drug will (usually) be more soluble in nonpolar solvents such as ether, benzene, or chloroform. These weak acid/weak base forms are easily interconverted by changing the pH:

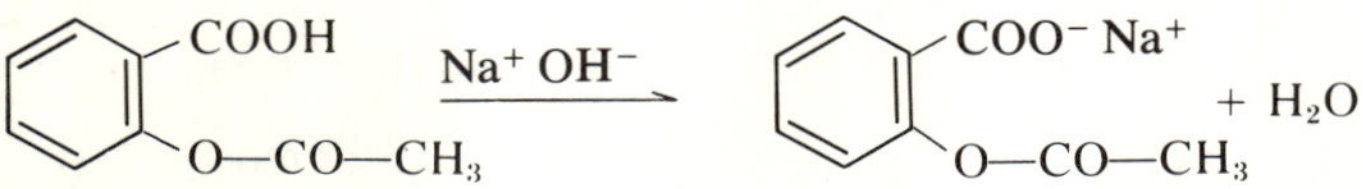

aspirin

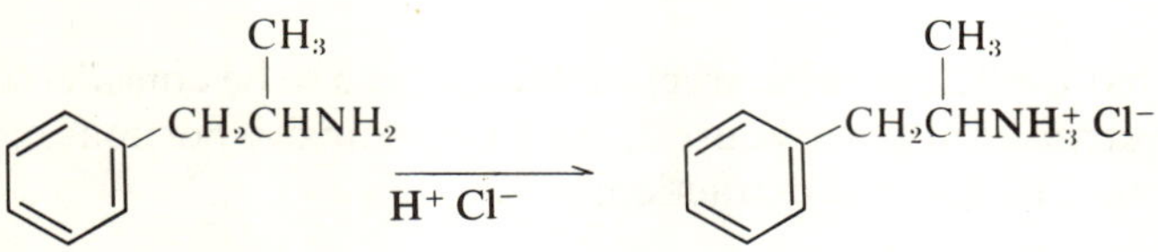

amphetamine

Remember that pH = pK_a + log [ionized form]/[unionized form] (p. 24). If the pK_a of a drug = 5.0, then

at pH = 5	50 percent will be in the ionized form
6	90
7	99
8	99.9

and it will be decreasingly extractable into nonpolar solvents as pH increases: i.e., the partition coefficients are pH-dependent for these compounds.

Advantage is taken of this in many analytical separations. Suppose we wished to determine both ephedrine and phenobarbital in combinations of both (e.g., Warner-Chilcott's Tedral preparations). Ephedrine hydrochloride is soluble in water; phenobarbital is not appreciably so. If we make an aqueous suspension of the mixture basic, ephedrine hydrochloride will be converted to the free base which is less soluble in water than the salt, whereas phenobarbital will be converted to its sodium salt which is much more water soluble. By any of the methods described above, the ephedrine may be extracted with ether and its concentration in the mixture determined.

Acidification of the aqueous phase will convert phenobarbital back to its unionized form; re-extraction of this mixture with ether will then recover this compound for its quantitative estimation. A flow diagram for such an assay might look like the one seen on p. 69. Similar extractions are used for many U.S.P. assays.

We have assumed that the concentrations of the separated phases could be determined by simple evaporation and weighing. In practice, more sophisticated methods are used, and much of the remainder of this text will concern itself with these.

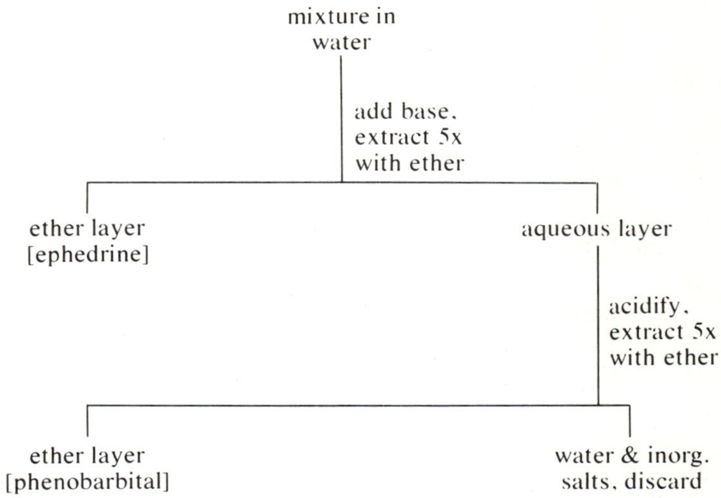

THINGS TO REMEMBER

$$K = C_1/C_2 \qquad U = V_1/V_2$$

$$p = KU/[KU + 1]$$

$$q = 1/[KU + 1]$$

Fraction remaining after n extractions $= q^n$
Total extracted after n extractions $= 1 - q^n$

Experiment 10. Determination of the Partition Coefficient of 8-Hydroxyquinoline

Students may work in pairs. Partition coefficients are to be determined in triplicate.

Stock Solution, 8-Hydroxyquinoline. Weigh out 145 mg. of 8-hydroxyquinoline and transfer it to a 1 L. volumetric flask. Fill the flask to mark with octanol-saturated deionized water (OSW). Pipet 10 ml. of this solution into a 100 ml. volumetric flask and fill to mark with OSW. This solution contains 1×10^{-4} M 8-hydroxyquinoline.

Standard Solutions. Samples of the stock solution are diluted by taking 10.0, 15.0, 20.0, and 25.0 ml. samples and placing them in 100 ml. volumetric flasks and filling with OSW to give a series of solutions ranging in concentration from 10^{-5} to 2.5×10^{-5} M. Place aliquots of each of these samples in an ultraviolet absorption cell and determine the absorption at 235 nm. When this is plotted against concentration, a straight line should result (see discussion of Beer's law, p. 99).

Determination of Partition Coefficient. A 50.0 ml. aliquot of the 2×10^{-5} M standard solution is placed in a 250 ml. flask and 50 ml. of octanol saturated with water is added. The mixture is shaken for 60 min. and allowed to stand so that the layers can separate. An aliquot of the water layer is placed in an ultraviolet cell and the absorption determined at 235 nm. From the standard curve, the concentration of 8-hydroxyquinoline in the water layer is determined. The concentration in the octanol layer is determined by subtracting that of the water layer from the initial concentration. The partition coefficient is then determined by:

$$K_d = \text{concentration in octanol/concentration in water}$$

PROBLEMS

1. A 25.00 ml. aliquot of a 0.4 percent (w/v) aqueous solution of acetanilid was extracted with three 10.00 ml. portions of ether. The combined ether extracts were evaporated to dryness and the residue was weighed. The ether/water partition coefficient for acetanilid is 3.000. What is the weight of the residue?
2. How many extractions are necessary to remove 99.9 percent of a drug from 50 ml. of an aqueous solution if it is extracted with 25 ml. portions of ether and its partition coefficient is 1.0?
3. The solubility of phenobarbital is given as 1.0 gm./100 ml. of water and 1.0 gm./13 ml. of ether. Using these data, calculate the approximate partition coefficient for phenobarbital in this system. Using this value for K, calculate the number of extractions necessary for 99.9 percent recovery of a sample of phenobarbital from a 100 mg. tablet using equal volumes (200 ml.) of water and ether.
4. A sample of powdered codeine phosphate tablets equivalent to 100 mg. of codeine phosphate was dissolved in 100 ml. of water, made alkaline with ammonia, and extracted three times with 20 ml. portions of ether. If the partition coefficient for codeine in the ether/water system is 8.0, how much codeine could be recovered? Mol. wt. codeine = 299.36, its phosphate salt (+1/2 H_2O) = 406.37.
5. Caffeine Sodium Benzoate Injection (U.S.P. XIX, 59) is a sterile solution containing approximately equal amounts of the two ingredients. A 2.0 ml. sample was transferred to a small separatory funnel and made alkaline with a drop of sodium hydroxide solution. The mixture was then extracted with a 20.0 ml. portion of chloroform. If 98.8 percent of the caffeine were extracted, calculate the K_d for this substance in the chloroform-water system.
6. The solubility of chloramphenicol is given as 2.5 mg./ml. in water, 0.25 mg./ml. in benzene, and 25 mg./ml. in ether. Which of the solvents would you use to extract chloramphenicol from its aqueous solutions? Why?

ANSWERS

1. 0.0906 gm.
2. 17 extractions
3. 4 extractions
4. 69.4 mg. codeine
5. 8.2

Chapter 9

Chromatography

Chromatography is a more elegant and more complicated technique for separation than the one we have just discussed, yet in many ways the concepts we have learned are applicable to this method also. The term chromatography literally means writing or drawing with color; the first compounds isolated by this method were plant pigments. The chlorophyll of green leaves is actually a mixture of chlorophylls which were separated from one another by the Russian scientist Tswett in 1906. Although the method was not widely used until about 25 years after its discovery, recent years have seen a rather extraordinary development of the technique, and it has become one of the standard, universally acceptable methods for the separation of complex mixtures, including mixtures of colorless compounds.

We might begin to understand the process by considering first a modification of our familiar partition system. Consider a column of one liquid (water) being extracted by a fine stream or spray of a second, immiscible liquid (chloroform) (see figure, p. 72). Apparatus designed for such extractions by liquids lighter or heavier than water is available. This obviates the need to shake separatory funnels; the liquid falling (or rising) through the aqueous layer extracts substances more soluble in it according to principles already learned. Now imagine two changes: (1) construct a column in which one of these liquids is held on some type of solid support; (2) pass a solution of a mixture of substances through this column at a rate which allows these substances to partition themselves between this liquid film and the solvents as the mixture passes through the column. It is not difficult to see that substances more soluble in the supported liquid (e.g., water)—*the stationary phase*—will distribute themselves into this liquid whereas others will simply flow through the column with the solvent—*the mobile phase*—and be collected at the lower end. Basically, this is *partition chromatography.* It depends, as does extraction, on the property of a substance which enables it to dissolve in one or another of the liquids involved.

A second property of substances which has a bearing on the success of this technique is the tendency to become attached to (adsorbed on) the surface of a finely divided solid. If the mobile phase is a liquid containing a mixture of substances, some of these, under appropriate conditions, will be preferentially adsorbed onto the stationary phase as the solution passes through the column. This is known as *adsorption chromatography.* Very often adsorption and partition take place at the same time in a given column.

Sometimes the mobile phase is a gas rather than a solvent which carries a volatile

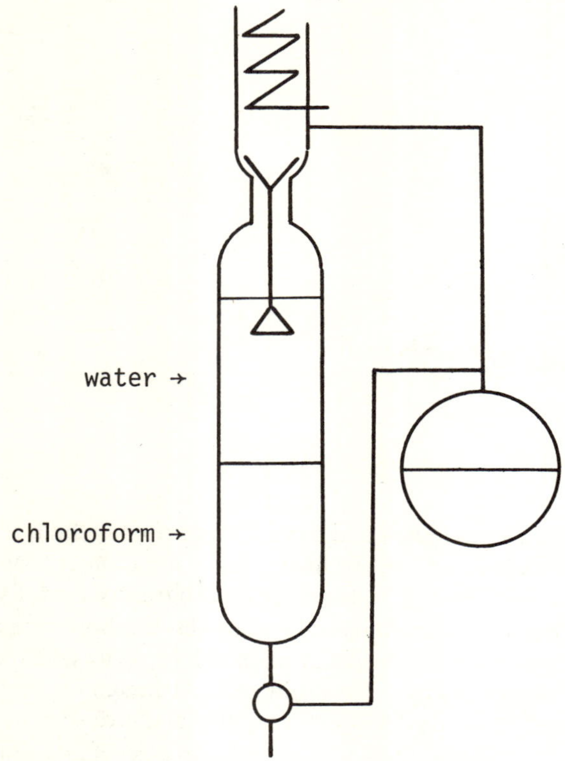

substance or mixture through the column. Mostly, but not always, the stationary phase is a liquid film on some supporting solid. This is called *vapor phase chromatography* or simply *gas chromatography* rather than its more complex name, gas-liquid-partition chromatography.

A few more terms will be helpful in the discussions which follow. A solid substance used as a stationary phase is called the *adsorbent*. The material holding a liquid film column is called the *support*. When a moving phase is caused to pass over these for the purpose of separation, the process is called *development*. Substances to be separated are called the *solutes* or *samples*. The solvent(s) in which they are dissolved (except in gas chromatography) is (are) known as the *solvent(s)* or *solvent system*. If substances are washed out of or off of the adsorbent, the process is called *elution*. The solution thus obtained is the *eluate*. Finally we will consider methods of *detection* particularly in cases where the substances eluted have insufficient color to be detected by the eye. Using these definitions, a brief survey of the commonly used techniques may be given.

Columm Chromatography

Whether adsorption or partition chromatography is used, the stationary phase is often silica, alumina, sugar, starch, charcoal, or cellulose. Other adsorbents are used for special applications. The mobile phase, at least at the beginning of a chromatogram, is the least polar solvent capable of dissolving the solutes to be separated. The figure on p. 73 represents the stages in the development of a typical chromatogram. Substance 1 is adsorbed/partitioned to a different degree than substance 2; it moves down the column more rapidly

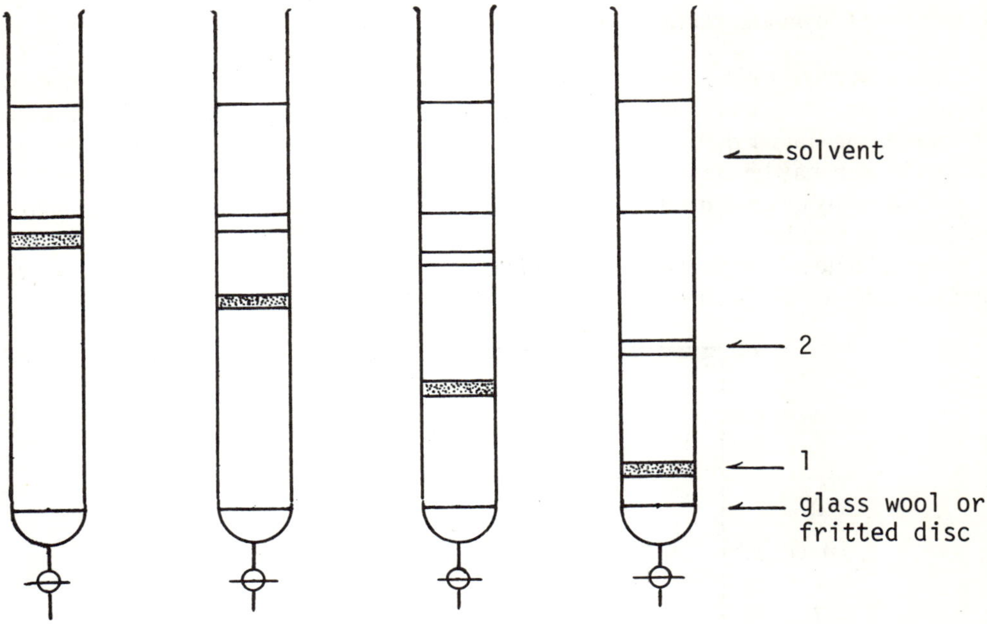

and hence becomes separated from 2. If this effect is visible, one might drain the column of solvent, extrude it, and cut the band of substance 1 from substance 2 and elute these separately with a more polar solvent. Very often it is not visible. In this event, it is possible to continue passage of solvent through the column until substance 1 is completely washed out. Evaporation of the eluate gives that substance followed later by the recovery of substance 2 in the same fashion. This is called *elution analysis*.

In most instances, it will be found that two substances, or a mixture of two or more, will not be separated so easily on a column using a single solvent for development. For example, substance 2 might not be eluted at all with the solvent used to elute substance 1. It is then necessary to modify (increase) the polarity of the solvent system in order to elute 2, e.g., by the addition of a small amount of alcohol to chloroform. The more substances in the mixture to be separated, the greater the number of increments of polarity that may have to be used to elute the substances serially. This is called *gradient elution analysis*.

We have mentioned a number of adsorbents that are useful in column chromatography. Alumina (Al_2O_3) is often used for amines or alkaloids, silica (SiO_2) for neutral or acidic compounds. These adsorbents can function as partition supports as well by the addition of small amounts of liquid, e.g., water. The general rule that the least polar solvent which will dissolve the solutes is the one chosen suggests that one might begin with petroleum ether, follow with the same solvent containing known increments of benzene, then with benzene itself, followed by benzene plus measured amounts of ether. This process continues until a highly polar solvent such as methanol might be used for the final elution. Columns are usually glass tubes 10 to 100 times as long as their internal diameter depending on the substances to be separated. The adsorbent is usually taken in an amount equal to 20 to 50 times the weight of the sample to be separated; for more complete separation, or with very complex mixtures, 200 to 2000 times the weight of the sample may be required. These rough guides are modified according to circumstances.

Thin Layer Chromatography (TLC)

If the adsorbing solid is prepared in the form of a thin layer (250 μ) on a glass plate or a plastic sheet, we are able to carry out chromatography on this layer rather than in a column, using similar theory and development. A number of points concerning the use of this technique may be mentioned.

1. Plates may be coated with the same adsorbents used for columns although usually the particles are smaller.

2. Small amounts (e.g., 2 to 5 μl.) of a 1 percent solution of a substance or a mixture are spotted at the origin (see figure below).

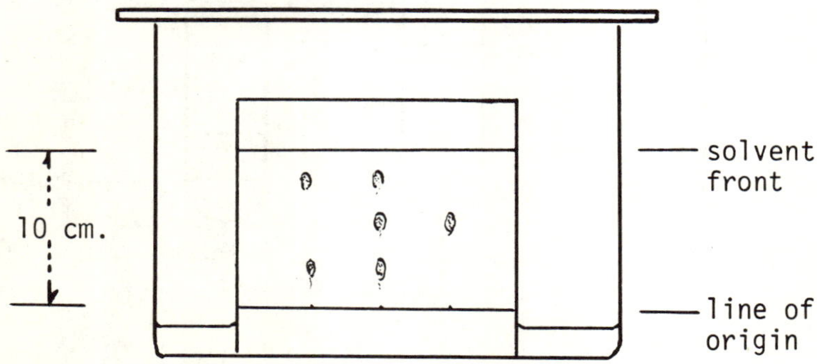

3. The plate is developed by enclosure in a chamber containing a solvent system appropriate to the substance(s) to be chromatographed and in an amount such that the level of the liquid comes just below the line of origin.

4. After development, the separated substances will be found as distinct spots at various distances from the line of origin. They may be detected by an appropriate reagent sprayed onto the plate or sometimes by their fluorescence in ultraviolet light.

$$R_f = \frac{\text{distance from origin to center of spot}}{\text{distance to front of developing solvent}}$$

Two substances which give identical R_f values when chromatographed under carefully controlled conditions in several solvent systems may be assumed identical.

5. TLC is subject to many variables: temperature, activity of the adsorbent, concentration of the sample spotted, distance from the solvent reservoir to the base line, equilibration of the vapor in the cabinet, movement of the tank during development. It is common practice when using this method as a means of identification to spot an authentic specimen of the suspected compound on the same plate so that R_f values can be compared critically after development.

Detection. Obviously if the substances to be separated are colorless, means of detection are necessary so that spots can be located and their R_f values measured. There are several ways to do this.

1. Spray reagents react with the substances on the sheet to form colored complexes, e.g., Ninhydrin with amino acids, Dragendorff's reagent with alkaloids, ferric chloride with phenols.

2. Ultraviolet light will cause some compounds to fluoresce and plates can be examined for this. Some compounds will quench fluorescence so that if the adsorbing layer has a

fluorescent substance incorporated in it, spots due to such compounds will show dark against a fluorescent background. R_f values are measured from the line of origin to the center of the spot, and the solvent front from the same line to the maximum distance the developer was allowed to run, usually 10 cm.

Two-Dimensional TLC.

Sometimes it is not possible to separate two substances with a single developing system; the R_f values are too nearly the same. One might then resort to two-dimensional TLC. The substances are spotted and developed in the usual fashion in one solvent system. The plate is then dried, turned 90°, and redeveloped in a second solvent system.

Paper Chromatography (PC).

This is analogous to a cellulose column; a layer of cellulose is applied to a plate or sheet as for TLC or, simply, a sheet of filter paper may be used. This too may be used for partition chromatography by impregnation with one solvent and development with another, or for adsorption chromatography. The mobile phase is usually a mixed solvent; it may be basic or acidic depending on the type of compounds to be separated. For example, isopropanol-ammonia-water or *n*-butanol-acetic acid-water are often used.

There are three main types of paper chromatography. (1) The sheet is lowered into the developer as for TLC and the solvent rises by capillary action. This is called ascending paper chromatography. As for TLC, the mobile phase passes over the sample, a distribution between phases occurs, and compounds with a greater affinity for the mobile phase migrate fastest. (2) Descending paper chromatography is based on the same principle but utilizes downward, gravity flow of the developing solvent. (3) In circular or radial chromatography, the sample is applied to the center of the paper supported across a dish or beaker and the developer is fed to the center by a wick. Concentric rings are produced instead of spots.

Gas Chromatography.

Basically this is column partition chromatography in which the mobile phase is an inert gas which carries the mixture through the column. The solid support, which may be packed into glass or stainless steel tubes, is usually an inert material impregnated with a polymeric liquid with a high boiling point. To maintain volatile compounds in the vapor state the entire apparatus is usually enclosed in an oven, the temperature of which can be regulated (see figure, p. 76).
The carrier gas may be He, Ar, N_2, or H_2; temperature may be programmed. The detector responds to the presence of anything but the carrier gas. The recorder is activated by the detector to indicate, on a moving chart, a signal that substances are coming off of the column. A time-signal plot may look like that shown in the figure on p. 76.

The detector indicates the presence of the various components and measures their relative concentrations as they come off the column. The two most common types involve (a) thermal conductivity, and (b) flame ionization.

The thermal conductivity detector operates on the principle that heat is transported away from a hot body at a rate which depends on its composition. In this case the hot body is the gas stream. The detector system uses two heated filaments. The sample plus carrier gas pass over one while the carrier gas alone passes over the other. The detector compares

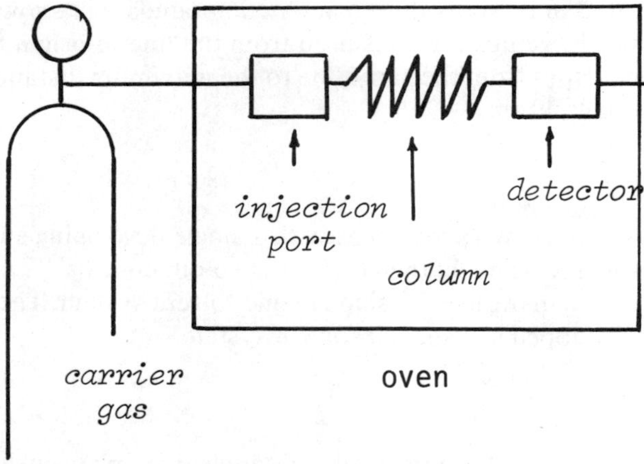

the thermal conductivity of the two and any differences result in peak formation. This method is nondestructive, e.g., the sample can be isolated after detection, but it is less sensitive than the flame ionization detector.

This latter device utilizes a flame produced by burning hydrogen to give rise to water. When an organic compound is present in the gas stream it, too, burns with the resulting formation of CO_2 the amount of which is measured. The sensitivity of the detector is proportional to the carbon content of the compound. The method obviously requires that a sample burn and that the sample is thereby destroyed.

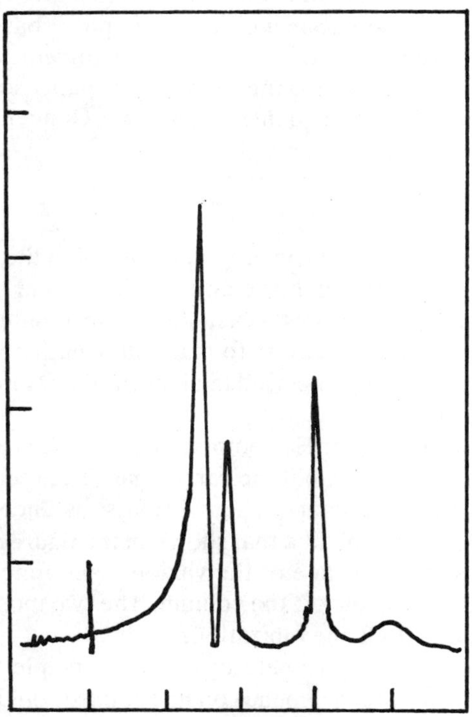

The retention time (R_t) is analogous to the R_f in other methods and is characteristic of a given substance under specified experimental conditions. By introduction of an internal standard of known concentration, the method can be made quantitative inasmuch as the area under the signal peak is proportional to the concentration of the substance.

The method has a number of advantages: (1) very small amounts of material can be detected, (2) the method can be used for separation by putting a cold trap in the line and catching the substances responsible for the recorded peaks as they come off of the column, (3) it can be used for the determination of the number of constituents in a mixture, and (4) it can be used as a measure of the purity of a sample. However, not all substances are easily separated by this technique. Special conditions may have to be devised for the separation of a mixture of substances which have nearly equal volatilities, and thus very similar retention times, or compounds which, because of very low volatility, take unduly long to move through columns even at relatively high temperatures or are liable to decomposition at these temperatures. In many cases these difficulties may be overcome by converting the compounds to derivatives. For example, steroids, after isolation from a urine sample, have been converted to their trimethylsilyl ethers which give much improved separation permitting easier identification and quantitative estimation. A similar device has been used for the determination of phenytoin, a process which is described on p. 81.

Ion-Exchange Chromatography

We often find that highly polar compounds, especially ionized species, are too strongly adsorbed on conventional columns, are nonvolatile, or are too insoluble in nonpolar solvents to permit separation by the methods so far discussed. Certain inorganic substances (e.g., zeolites) and a group of synthetic resins in particular have, as part of their structures, groups at the surface of their particles capable of exchanging ions with the medium in which they are placed. There are two major types:

1. *Cation exchangers* are polymers with COOH or SO_3H groups which can exchange with other cations.

$$R{-}SO_3^-\,H^+ + Na^+ \rightarrow R{-}SO_3^-\,Na^+ + H^+$$

2. *Anion exchangers* are polymers having $R{-}NH_3^+\,OH^-$ or $R{-}N(CH_3)_3^+\,OH^-$ groups capable of exchanging with other anions.

$$RNH_3^+\,OH^- + Cl^- \rightarrow RNH_3^+\,Cl^- + OH^-$$

In both cases, R is a polymeric resin moiety. Depending on the formulation of the resin, these columns can also act as adsorbents as in other column procedures.

There are a number of pharmaceutical applications of the method:

1. Deionization of water (containing NaCl, $MgCl_2$, Na_2SO_4, etc.):

(a) Adsorb cations on a cation exchanger.

$$R{-}SO_3^-\,H^+ + MX \rightarrow R{-}SO_3^-\,M^+ + H^+ + X^-$$

(b) Adsorb anions on an anion exchanger.

$$R{-}NH_3^+\,OH^- + HX \rightarrow R{-}NH_3^+\,X^- + OH^- + H^+$$

The net result is pure water.

2. Analysis of salt solutions:

$$R—SO_3^- H^+ + KNO_3 \rightarrow R—SO_3^- K^+ + H^+ + NO_3^-$$

The column may be washed with water and the nitric acid titrated with standard base.

3. Concentration of ions from dilute solution (hardness tests) may be accomplished by adsorption of trace ions. The volume chosen to elute them is less than the original volume, and the ions can be determined by the usual methods.

4. Good separation of amino acids can be achieved by ion-exchange chromatography.

5. Many drug screening tests depend on the adsorption of the drugs from urine or blood onto ion-exchange columns, followed by elution with buffers at specified pH and determination of the drugs separately. Morphine, amphetamines, and barbiturates are often detected in this way.

High-Pressure Liquid Chromatography

A method which overcomes the problem of poorly volatile compounds in gas chromatography, including many pharmaceutical agents, has found increasing use during the last few years. This is *high-pressure* or *high-performance liquid chromatography (HPLC)*. In principle it is similar to gas chromatography. The instrument includes a pump to force the mobile phase through the column, an injection system for introduction of the sample, a column, a detector, and a recorder.

The columns used for HPLC are made of glass or, more often, metal and may be packed with a variety of adsorbents including silica of 5μ or smaller particle size or polymeric substances bonded to a solid support. The mobile phase is driven through the column at pressures ranging from 500 to 5000 lbs./in.^{2} A constant pressure is important for reproducible retention times, peak heights, and peak areas necessary for quantitative estimation. Three techniques for sample injection are commonly used. Syringe injection involves the use of a septum and allows for easy variation in sample size, but repeated injections at higher pressures may result in leakage at the septum which will produce variations in peak height and peak symmetry. Sample-loop injection allows for greater precision and eliminates the need for constant replacement of septa. It involves the use of a plastic tube that is filled with solvent which is then released into the column. Leaks seen with syringe injection do not occur. When the instrument is run at very high pressures, the stop-flow injection method is used. The solvent flow is stopped, a pressure guard over the septum is removed, the sample is injected, the septum guard replaced, and the solvent flow resumed. The procedure is simple but time-consuming.

The detectors used in HPLC are generally less sensitive than those available for gas chromatographs. Detectors found on commercial instruments utilize differences in the ultraviolet absorption or the refractive index of the fractions being eluted from the column.

Three papers recently published in the *Journal of Pharmaceutical Sciences* illustrate the application of this method to pharmaceutical problems. They deal with the detection of pilocarpine and isopilocarpine in pharmaceutical preparations,* the determination of procaine,† and the determination of theophylline in plasma.‡

Gel Chromatography

One other technique which has found wide application in the separation of substances such as carbohydrates, proteins, and lipids is that of gel chromatography, sometimes called exclusion chromatography. By this method it is possible to separate mixtures on the basis of the molecular weights of their constituents. It differs from adsorption chromatography in a number of ways. In place of a stationary phase held on a solid support, it utilizes carbohydrate, styrene, or acrylamide polymers prepared in such a way as to give regular cross-linked structure. When the polymers are soaked in water or other solvents, swelling occurs which results in the formation of channels through the polymers. By specific manufacturing processes, various grades of these gels can be prepared based on their ability to take up water. There is a relationship between the grade and the size of the molecules (range of molecular weights) able to permeate the gel, leading to separation of the constituents of the mixtures applied to the column. Thus, when a mixture containing both small and large molecules is put on such a column, the smaller molecules permeate the gel and are retarded in their movement down the column. Compounds of larger molecular weight are not able to enter the gel matrix and therefore pass through the column as readily as the solvent. The various types of gels differ in their physical and chemical characteristics. Carbohydrate polymers are hydrolyzed by strong acid and are subject to bacterial or fungal attack which may limit their use in certain applications. Polystyrene gels cannot be used with water and alcohols but are useful for nonaqueous separations. The polyacrylamides are stable over a pH range from about 2 to 12, but since they do not contain the numerous hydroxy groups of the carbohydrate gels, they are not suitable for the separation of polar substances.

Experiment 11. Chromatography

Thin-Layer Chromatographic Identification of the Major Alkaloids of *Cinchona Bark*

About 40 alkaloids have been isolated from the genus *Cinchona* but not all of them have a demonstrated medicinal importance. The presence of any given alkaloid in detectable amounts depends on many factors, including the species examined, its origin, the part of the plant examined, etc. In the following experiment at least three alkaloids should be identifiable under the conditions described.

1. Moisten about 100 mg. of the powdered plant material in a test tube with two drops of 25 percent aqueous ammonia solution. Add 5 ml. of chloroform, cork the tube, and shake for about 10 min. Filter through a small plug of glass wool into a clean test tube, and wash

---

*Urbanyi, T., et al.: *Simultaneous determination of pilocarpine and isopilocarpine in pharmaceutical preparations by liquid chromatography.* J. Pharm. Sci. 65:275, 1976.

†Wahba Khalil, S. K., and Shelver, W. H.: *High-speed liquid chromatographic determination of procaine in pharmaceuticals.* J. Pharm. Sci. 65:606, 1976.

‡Weddle, O. H., and Mason, W. D.: *Rapid determination of theophylline in human plasma by high-pressure liquid chromatography.* J. Pharm. Sci. 65:865, 1976.

the plant material on the filter with a small portion of fresh chloroform. Evaporate the combined filtrates and washings to dryness on the water bath (hood!) using an applicator stick to prevent bumping. After cooling, take up the residue in 1 ml. of methanol and set this extract aside. Take a silica gel sheet and with a pencil (not a pen) mark a light line 1 cm. from one edge. With this line at the bottom, place marks at the left and right edges of the sheet 10 cm. from the base line. Now spot 5 μl. of your plant extract on the base line at least 1 cm. in from the edge of the sheet. Keep the spot as small as possible. About 1 cm. from it, spot 2 μl. of the standard alkaloid solution provided. At least four students can spot solutions on the same plate. Place the plate in the developing tank containing a mixture of benzene:ether:diethylamine = 55:35:10 and allow the solvent to rise to the 10 cm. mark. Remove the plate and allow it to dry for 10 min. in a stream of dry air at room temperature. A hair dryer is useful for this purpose. Return it to the tank and develop it again to the 10 cm. mark.

2. While development of the plate is in progress, evaporate the remainder of the methanolic extract to dryness in the water bath. Add a drop of glacial acetic acid to the residue, then a drop of distilled water. With a glass rod spot a drop of this solution onto a piece of filter paper. Moisten it with a drop of Dragendorff's reagent. Note the result. To the remainder, add 2.5 ml. of 4 N sulfuric acid and an equal volume of distilled water. Shake for a minute and filter. To 1 ml. of the filtrate, add a few drops of Mayer's reagent and note the result. Examine the rest of the solution in long-wavelength ultraviolet (UV) light. Describe the result.

3. When development of the plate is complete, remove it and dry it in an oven at 100°C. to volatilize the diethylamine in the solvent. Cool and examine the plate under short-wavelength UV light. With a sharp instrument (dissecting needle or sharp pencil point) mark the centers of any distinct spots which you observe, and note their colors.

4. Spray the plate with the methanol-sulfuric acid solution and examine it under long-wavelength UV light. Do the spots correspond to those you observed previously? Note their colors.

5. Now spray the plate with the iodoplatinate reagent. If the centers of the spots visualized by this method do not correspond to those marked previously, mark any new spot. Measure the R_f values (see p. 74) of the substances in the standard solution, then of those in the plant sample. The intensity and size of the spots is a rough measure of the concentration of the substances in the mixture. While the R_f values depend on a number of factors, in this experiment the following values may be anticipated: quinine, 0.25 to 0.35; cinchonidine, 0.40 to 0.50; and cinchonine 0.60 to 0.70.

Gas Chromatographic Analysis of Dilute Alcohol Solutions

This experiment is adapted from that of Parker and coworkers.* A column of 60 to 80 mesh Chromosorb-W, acid washed and coated with 40 percent Castorwax should be preconditioned (190°C., 8 hr.) before use. Operating conditions should be: injector temperature, 170°C., oven temperature, 120°C.; N_2 gas stream at 13.6 ml./min.; volume injected, 1 μl.; attenuation, 8 times; flame ionization detector. Microsyringes should be washed approximately 10 times with distilled water between injections. Aqueous solutions of methanol, ethanol, or isopropanol will serve as unknowns. Your sample may contain

*Parker, K. D., et al.: *Gas chromatographic determination of ethyl alcohol in blood for medicolegal purposes.* An. Chem. 34:1234, 1962.

more than one of the alcohols mentioned. Each unknown will also contain a known concentration of butanol as an internal standard to facilitate calculation of the concentration of the unknown alcohol.

Inject 2 μl. of your sample into the gas chromatograph. Compare the retention times for your peaks with those of standard samples previously run by the laboratory instructor, and identify the unknown(s) in your sample. Measure peak heights of your alcohol(s) and of butanol, the internal standard. The concentration of your sample may be determined by using the following equation:

$$\text{concentration of unknown} = \frac{\text{peak height of unknown}}{\text{peak height of internal standard}} \times \text{concentration of internal standard}$$

This relationship does not exist for all determinations, but it has been experimentally verified for the unknowns and the internal standard used in this particular experiment.

Gas Chromatographic Assay of Phenytoin in Blood Serum

In many clinical analyses, the techniques of solvent extraction and chromatography are used in combination. An example of this is the measurement of blood levels of phenytoin, a drug widely used in the treatment and control of epilepsy and other convulsive disorders. Since there are great differences between individuals in the metabolism of the drug, it sometimes requires monitoring of the blood levels to allow adjustments of the dose and thus to decrease the occurrence of side effects in a particular patient. These may include depression, hyperplasia of the gums, tremor, and dermatitis. The older chemical methods for the assay of phenytoin are very tedious, requiring as long as 4 hr. to complete. They are also subject to interference by phenobarbital or other barbiturates which may be administered with phenytoin. The solvent extraction-gas chromatographic method now used in some laboratories has the advantage of being both rapid and accurate.

1. Prepare standard solutions of phenytoin containing 5, 10, and 25 μg./ml.
2. To 1 ml. of each standard and to a 1 ml. serum sample, add 1 ml. of 1 N HCl and 7 ml. of chloroform. Shake to extract; remove and discard the water layer which contains basic compounds.
3. Add 5 ml. of 0.45 N NaOH. Shake to extract; discard the chloroform layer containing neutral compounds.
4. To the NaOH layer, add 1 ml. of 6N HCl and 10 ml. of chloroform; extract.
5. Draw off the chloroform layer and evaporate to dryness.
6. Dissolve the residue in 0.25 ml. of 0.2 M trimethylaniline hydroxide and inject 5 μl. of the mixture into the gas chromatograph (3 percent OV-17 on "Gas-chrom," T = 250°, flame ionization detector).

The following equations describe the process.

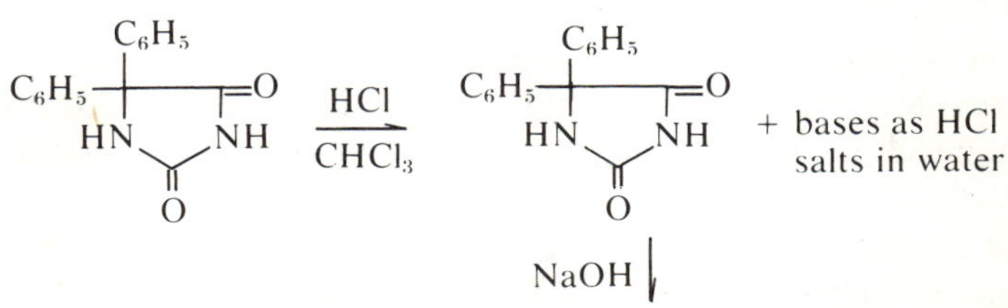

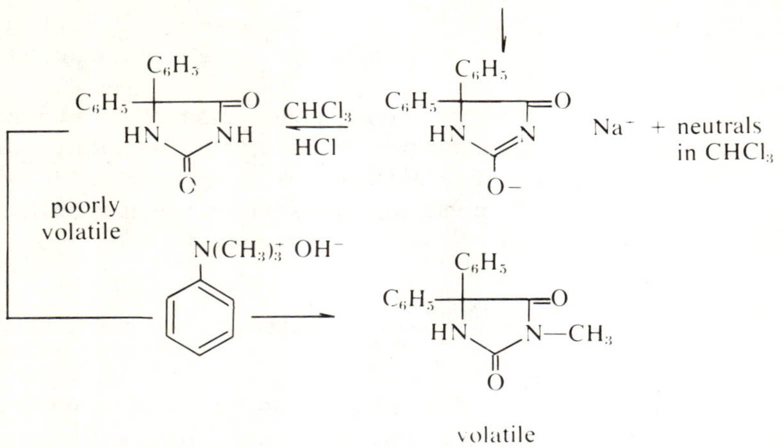

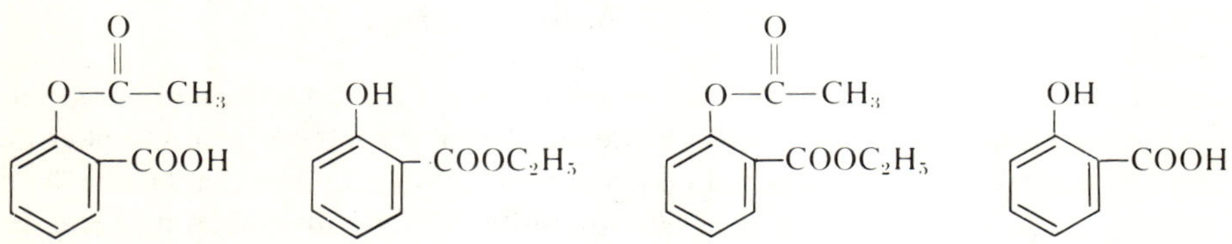

Thus, the extraction procedure eliminates all organic compounds but the acidic ones and the subsequent gas chromatographic analysis eliminates interference by other drugs such as barbiturates and aspirin. Comparing the peaks for the three standards allows calculation of the level of phenytoin in the blood.

PROBLEMS

1. List and define the various terms used to describe the types and techniques of solvent extraction and chromatography.
2. Explain how chromatographic techniques can be used for the concentration of substances from dilute solutions.
3. Explain why the R_f values for a given compound may not be strictly reproducible by TLC procedures from day to day. What steps would you take to eliminate these sources of error?
4. Outline a method for the identification and determination of (a) menthol in cigarette tobacco and (b) methyl salicylate in a sample supposed to be oil of wintergreen.
5. Outline a procedure for the quantitative analysis of each substance in a mixture of sodium bromide, phenobarbital, and phenytoin. Assume you have a sufficient amount of sample for your purpose.
6. Most caffeine in pharmaceutical use is prepared synthetically. Samples isolated from natural sources (e.g., tea) may contain related alkaloids (e.g., theophylline). Describe how you might identify the presence of this substance in a sample of caffeine of unknown origin.
7. Aspirin and the following derivatives of aspirin are to be separated by column chromatography. Predict their order of elution.

8. A patient was suspected of morphine addiction. A sample (20 ml.) of urine was available. Outline how you would detect the presence of morphine ($pK_a = 9.3$) in the sample.

Chapter 10

Optical Methods

Refractometry

Light, which we will consider from other points of view later, may be considered as electromagnetic radiation travelling as a wave from the source. The velocity or speed with which it travels depends on the medium through which it passes. Sunlight travels at different speeds through the vacuum of outer space, the earth's atmosphere, and urban smog. For practical purposes, we will consider only light passing through air and some other medium whose effect on light we wish to study. If the velocity changes with the medium, then in passing from one medium to another, a ray of light becomes bent, that is, it is said to be refracted (see figure below). A familiar example of this effect is the distortion

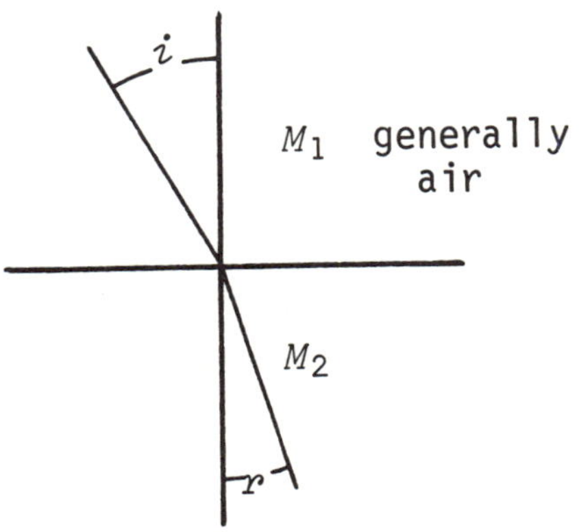

observed when a stick is immersed in a pool of water. The degree to which this bending takes place is called the *index of refraction* (n). It is described by the following relationships:

Eq. 1 $$n_{\lambda}^{t} = V_{M_1}/V_{M_2}$$

where t = temperature, λ = wavelength, V = velocity and M = medium. If i = the angle of incidence and r = the angle of refraction, it can be shown that

Eq. 2 $$n = \sin i/\sin r$$

as long as i is not equal to zero and M_1 and M_2 are different. This is known as *Snell's law.*

The index of refraction is a physical property of substances which can be used for their characterization. It is particularly applicable to liquids including many of pharmaceutical importance. However, the index of refraction of organic liquids is quite sensitive to changes in temperature. Routine measurements have a reproducibility of ±0.0002 units; an increase of 1°C. may result in changes of 0.0004 to 0.0005 units. Therefore temperature control is important. The wavelength of the light used is also important since n changes with λ also. This is controlled by use of a monochromatic light source, usually a sodium vapor lamp which emits the so-called "D-line" of Na at 583.9 nm. Unless otherwise specified, this light source is assumed.

The calculations necessary to establish the principles of optics based on light refraction are derived for a single ray of light. In practice it is not possible to isolate a single ray of light with which to make measurements; we have to deal, rather, with a beam, relatively broad, composed of many individual rays. One instrument used to determine n is called the Abbe refractometer. In principle, it consists of two halves of a prism between which a thin layer of the liquid sample is placed. A beam of light is reflected through the lower half of the prism, through the liquid, and finally into the upper half of the prism at the maximum angle of incidence (i.e., approximately 90° to the boundary normal, see figure, p. 85) which produces a maximal angle of refraction. The effect produced is observable through a small telescope. One part of the field may appear dark, the other light, or the field may appear wholly dark or light, depending on the position of the telescope with respect to the boundary. The reflector is moved until the field is half dark and half light, the cross hairs of the telescope being centered on the boundary between the two *(the critical boundary).* The angle through which the reflector must be moved to accomplish this is known as the *critical angle of refraction,* a measure of the refractive index. A scale on the instrument is calibrated so that this can be read directly. The principle is illustrated in the figure below. In practice, white light is used with a built-in optical compensator so that readings correspond to n_D. The prism is kept at constant temperature (usually 20 or 25°C.) by water circulated from a thermostatically controlled bath. The instrument may be calibrated by using pure water which has n_D = 1.3334 at 15°C.; 1.3330 at 20°C.; 1.3325 at 25°C. Any correction factor

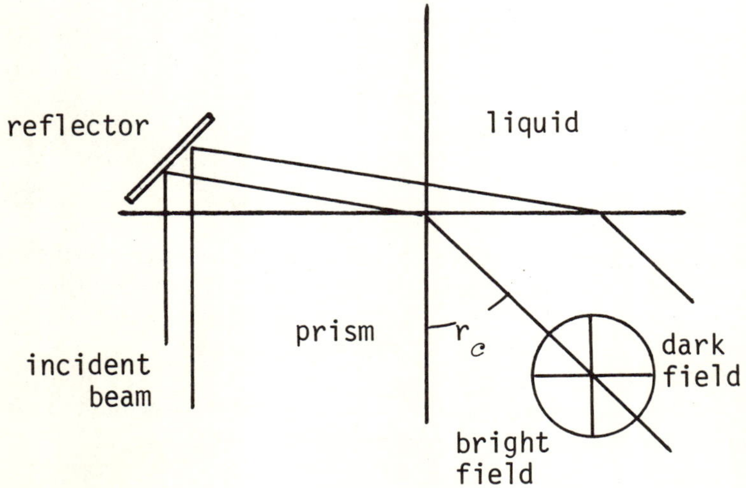

observed to be necessary should be applied to subsequent observations. Some instruments are supplied with a calibrating prism for the same purpose.

The method has several analytical applications.

1. The index of refraction is often used as a criterion for the identification of or purity of liquids, e.g., Eugenol (U.S.P. XIX, 193) has $n_D^{20°} = 1.540$ to 1.542.

2. The composition of mixtures of liquids used in pharmaceutical preparations (e.g., glycerol-water) may be established by determination of the index. Mixtures of known concentrations are prepared, and n_D is plotted against concentration. The composition of an unknown mixture may then be read directly from this graph when its index has been determined.

3. Rapid distinctions between similar substances are often possible by this method as can be seen:

Peanut oil	1.4625 – 1.4645 (40°)
Poppy seed oil	1.4766 – 1.4774 (20°)
Olive oil	1.4657 – 1.4667 (20°)
Peppermint oil	1.4590 – 1.4650 (20°)
Spearmint oil	1.4840 – 1.4910 (20°)
Clove oil	1.5270 – 1.5350 (20°)
Eugenol	1.5400 – 1.5420 (20°)

Note that the index of refraction for naturally occurring oils is often given as a range of values because the chemical composition of the plant oils varies with the origin, season harvested, soil conditions, climate, etc. of the plant from which they were derived.

POLARIMETRY

Using the concept that light consists of electromagnetic waves, we can assume a point source and see that the waves travelling out from this source will, if not impeded, travel in all directions and vibrate in all planes. If we were able to look at such a ray of light head on, the traces of the waves might look something like the diagram below. Such light is said to be unpolarized. It is possible to filter out light vibrating in all planes but one; this is then called *plane* or *linearly polarized light*. There are several ways in which light may be polarized:

1. Light is partially polarized by reflection. The glare of reflected sunlight on a bright day is partially polarized light.

2. Certain organic crystals do it. Iodoquinine crystals in Polaroid type sunglasses are used to filter out partially polarized light.

3. Some inorganic substances such as calcite ($CaCO_3$) will also do it.

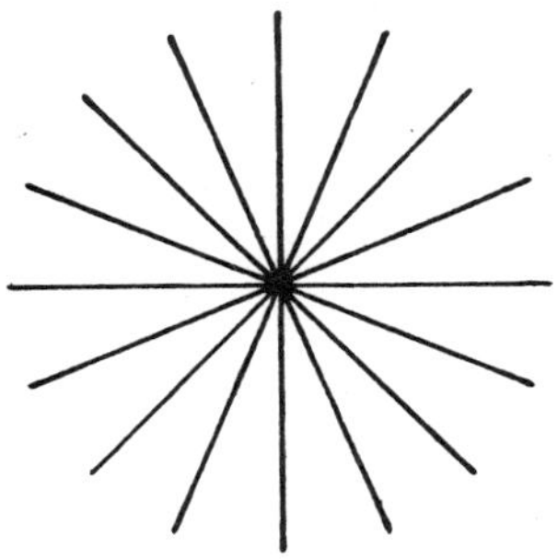

Without concern for the physics of the situation, we will accept the fact that two prisms of, for example, calcite can be cemented together in such a way that unpolarized light entering at one end of the system will emerge at the other end vibrating in one plane only, i.e., polarized. This is diagrammed below.

As you probably know, many organic substances, including many used as drugs, are said to be optically active, that is, they have the ability to rotate the plane of polarized light. If they do so to the left, they are said to be *levorotatory;* if to the right, *dextrorotatory.* Both the direction of rotation and the degree of rotation are characteristic for a pure substance. Thus, if we can measure this property, we have another criterion for the identity of and purity of that substance.

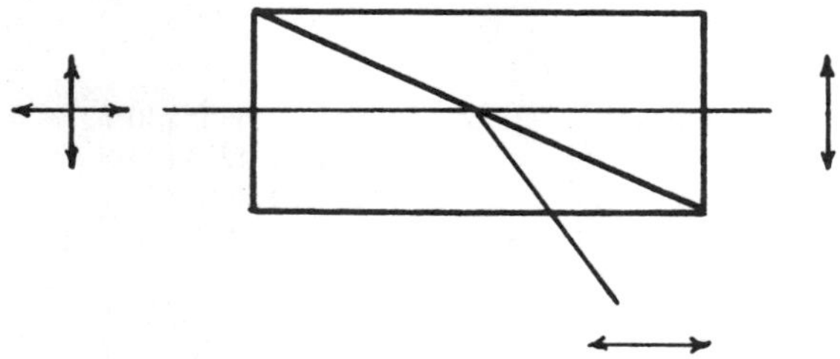

An instrument for the purpose, such as that shown below, can be imagined. L = a light source, P = a fixed polarizing prism, T = a tube for the sample, A = an analyzing prism identical to P but rotatable about the axis of the system, and O = the observer. Now, if the analyzer is set to match the polarizer, the exit beam from P will go directly through A to O and the field visible at O will be bright. If A is rotated 90°, the beam from P will be blocked out and the observed field will be dark. However, if we put a substance in T which is capable of rotating the plane of the polarized light coming from P, the plane of vibration of the light coming from A will be neither parallel to nor perpendicular to the vibration plane of the beam from P, and the observed field will be neither all dark nor all bright. We can then rotate A through some angle in order to restore either total darkness or maximum brightness, and this angle corresponds to the degree of rotation of the substance in T. The following relationships hold:

Eq. 3 $$[\alpha]^{t}_{\lambda} = 100\alpha/1c$$

where $[\alpha]$ = specific rotation
α = observed rotation
t = temperature
λ = wavelength of light used
l = length of tube in decimeters
c = concentration of substance in gm./100 ml.

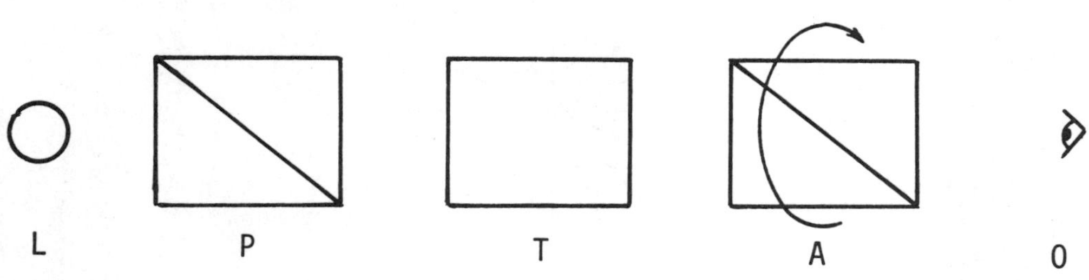

The direction of rotation is indicated by (+) if it is dextrorotation (to the right) or (−) if it is levorotation (to the left). The solvent used for the substance should be specified because values for optical rotation vary with the solvent. A typical citation might be given as $[\alpha]_D^{25} = -101°$ (c = 1, EtOH). For pure liquids not in solution (neat) a different expression is used:

Eq. 4 $$[\alpha]_\lambda^t = \alpha/ld \qquad \text{where } d = \text{density}$$

Sometimes it is desirable to compare compounds on the basis of their rotatory power using the expression for *molecular rotation:*

Eq. 5 $$[M]_\lambda^t = \alpha M/lc \qquad \text{where } M = \text{molecular weight}$$

The observed rotation also varies with the wavelength of the light used to measure it. This variation is called the *optical rotatory dispersion (ORD)* which has become a powerful tool in the elucidation of molecular configuration, but we will not have occasion to use it in this course.

For many of you, application of the technique of optical rotation to drug molecules will be a review of things learned in organic chemistry. Recall that the valence bonds of the carbon atom can be conceived as being directed to the corners of a tetrahedron (see figure below). When four different substituents are attached to this carbon atom, *two* different

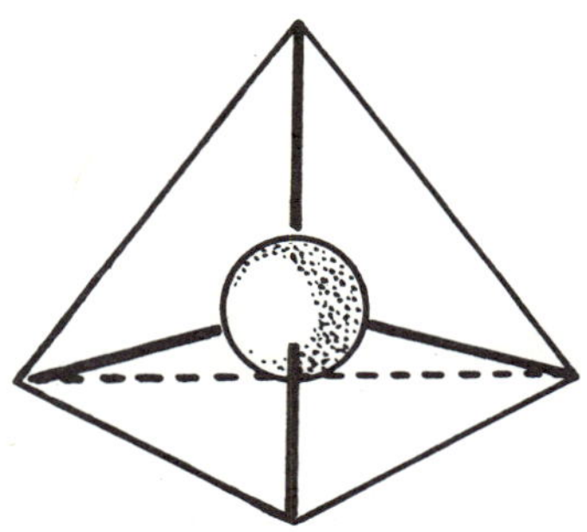

compounds result. These compounds are called *stereoisomers*. Let us represent the four corners of this tetrahedron by simpler planar diagrams (see below) and use as an example the amino acid alanine. If the C-atom is considered to be in the plane of the paper, those groups indicated with a broken line are to be considered to lie below that plane while those indicated with a solid line are to be thought of as lying above it. What makes these compounds different?

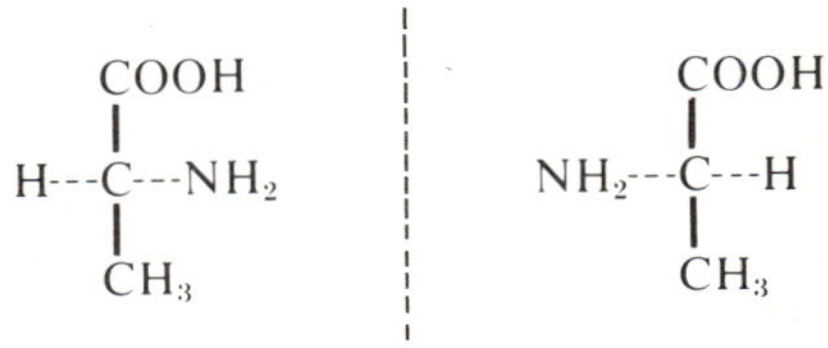

They are *mirror images* and *nonsuperimposable*. There is no way you can turn them around to superimpose one on the other without taking them out of the plane of the paper. Such a carbon atom is an *asymmetric* carbon atom, and such stereoisomers are called *enantiomers*.

All physical properties of these two compounds are alike, melting point, solubility, K_a, etc., EXCEPT optical activity. One will rotate the plane of polarized light to the right, the other to the left to the same degree.

Now consider a compound with two asymmetric carbon atoms alike in that each has the same four groups attached to it.

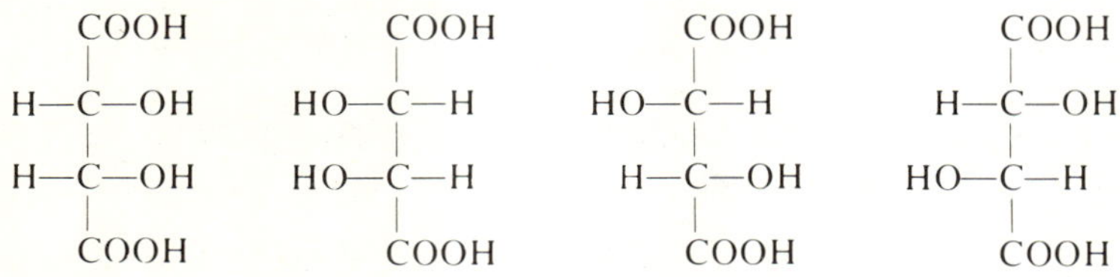

1 2 3 4

tartaric acid

Structures 1 and 2 are indeed mirror images, but they are superimposable by rotating one of them 180° in the plane of the paper. They are NOT enantiomers and therefore have no optical rotation. This is called the *meso* form of tartaric acid. Structures 3 and 4 are also mirror images, but they are not superimposable by any simple rotation. Hence these are enantiomers; one is dextrorotatory, the other levorotatory; the degree of rotation is equal but opposite. Note, however, that an equimolar mixture of the two will not rotate the plane of polarized light. Such a mixture is called *racemic* tartaric acid (± or *dl*). It can be separated into its two optically active components; a mixture of structures 1 and 2 cannot as they are not optically active.

As a final example, consider two unlike carbon atoms such as those in the four-carbon sugars.

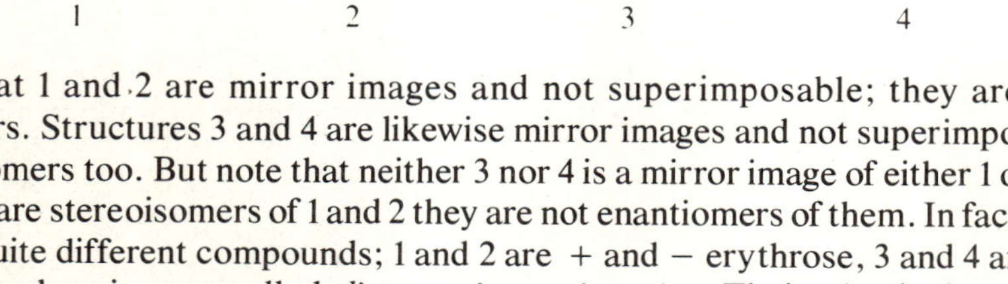

1 2 3 4

We see that 1 and 2 are mirror images and not superimposable; they are therefore enantiomers. Structures 3 and 4 are likewise mirror images and not superimposable; they are enantiomers too. But note that neither 3 nor 4 is a mirror image of either 1 or 2. Hence, while they are stereoisomers of 1 and 2 they are not enantiomers of them. In fact, these two pairs are quite different compounds; 1 and 2 are + and − erythrose, 3 and 4 are + and − threose. Such pairs are called *diastereoisomeric pairs*. Their physical and chemical properties are quite different.

We can conclude this discussion by mentioning some applications of the method:

1. Especially when combined with other data, it can establish a criterion for the identity and purity of a sample.

2. Correlation with biological activity of stereoisomeric compounds is possible because of the specificity of enzyme surfaces or reactive sites.

3. Since $\alpha = Kc$, the method can be used for the quantitative analysis of pure

compounds. This is especially true in sugar chemistry where the special term *saccharimetry* has been coined.

THINGS TO REMEMBER

$$n_\lambda^t = V_{M_1}/V_{M_2} = \sin i/\sin r$$

$$[\alpha]_\lambda^t = 100\alpha/lc$$

Experiment 12. Optical Methods

Polarimetry

The specific rotation of a substance can be used for its identification and as a criterion for its purity if the substance is optically active. In solution, the concentration of the compound and the nature of the solvent will determine the observed rotation as will the wavelength of the light used, the solution path, and the temperature. The equation by which the specific rotation can be calculated was given on p. 88.

Weigh accurately 10.0 gm. of your unknown substance and place it into a 100 ml. volumetric flask. Add water to dissolve and when solution is complete, make the final adjustment to volume. Fill a clean, dry observation tube with the solution avoiding air bubbles. Determine the value of the observed rotation by rotating the circular scale until the halves of the field, when viewed through the telescope, match in color intensity. Take at least three, and preferably five to seven, readings and calculate the mean. Do the same for a blank (water) and apply any necessary correction to the readings for your unknown sample. Using the corrected value, calculate the specific rotation of your unknown. The polarimeter tube may be cleaned by washing it with water followed by alcohol and ether. Your unknown substance will be from the following list: +20.5 to 21.5° (ascorbic acid); +72° (glucose); 103–105° (sodium ascorbate); +65.5–67° (sucrose).

Determination of Refractive Index

The refractive index of a substance is the ratio of the velocity of light in air to the velocity of light in the substance. It is valuable in the identification of substances such as the flavor and odor constituents of pharmaceutical preparations and often in the detection of impurities in such substances. It has also been used for determination of the composition of glycerol-water mixtures and the quantity of isopropanol in rubbing alcohol.

Place 2 or 3 drops of one of the oils supplied on the prism of the refractometer maintained at 25°C. with a water bath and clamp the prism together firmly. Fix the light source so that light is reflected through the prism, and adjust the instrument until the border line between the light and dark halves of the field coincides exactly with the cross-hairs of the telescope. Read the refractive index of the oil directly from the graduated scale.

The oils which you will be supplied as "unknowns" will be from the following list:

Clove oil	1.5270–1.5350
Eugenol	1.5400–1.5420
Lemon oil	1.4738–1.4755
Peppermint oil	1.4590–1.4650
Isopropyl alcohol	1.3763–1.3780

Make at least three determinations of the refractive index of your sample and report the mean value.

PROBLEMS

1. Define: plane polarized light, refractive index, optical activity, asymmetric carbon atom, enantiomers, stereoisomers, specific rotation, racemic modification, meso form, critical angle of refraction.
2. Explain all the terms in the following expressions, giving the units in which they are expressed:

$$n_D^t = \sin i/\sin r \qquad [\alpha]_\lambda^t = 100\alpha/lc$$

3. How would you distinguish between a and b if $n_D^{20°}$ of one does not differ by more than 0.0002 from the other?

(a) 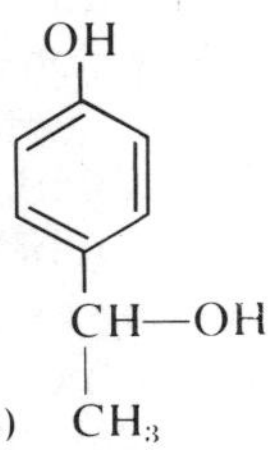

(b) 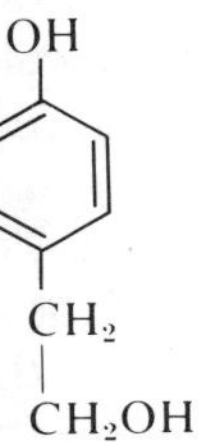

4. Cycloserine is represented by the following structure. Explain why it should show optical activity (+116° in water).

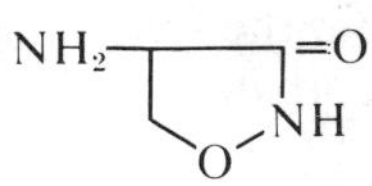

5. Five gm. of hyoscyamine was dissolved in chloroform to make 50.0 ml. The observed optical rotation in a 2 dm. tube at 20°C. using the sodium D-line was −5.04°. What is the specific rotation of hyoscyamine?

ANSWERS

5. −25.2°

Chapter 11

Visible, Ultraviolet, and Fluorescence Spectroscopy

We have defined light as electromagnetic radiation in the form of waves propagated by a source traveling through a medium.

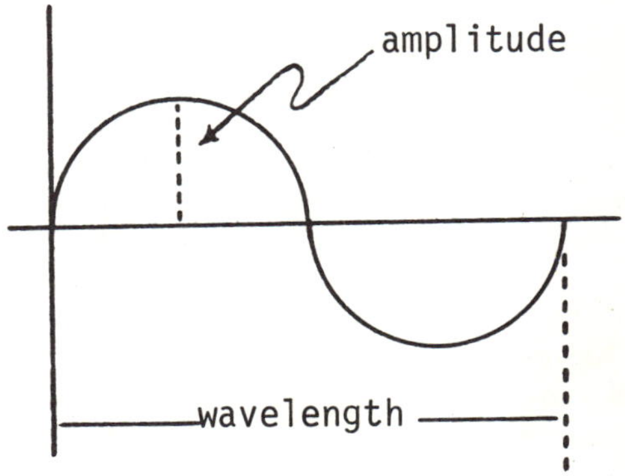

These waves have *energy* (electron volts, e.v.), *frequency* (ν) = number/unit time such as cycles/seconds (cps.) or Hertz (Hz.) or sometimes wave number ($1/\lambda$). They have a *wavelength* (λ) and an *amplitude* or maximum displacement. The frequency is related to the speed (velocity) and the wavelength.

Eq. 1 $$\nu = c/\lambda$$

where $c = 3 \times 10^{10}$ cm./sec., the speed of light in vacuum.

The range of radiations so far known and measured is termed the *electromagnetic spectrum* (Table 2). Several portions of this spectrum are important to the chemist.

All molecules possess energy by reason of: (1) moving from place to place (*translational*), (2) atoms moving with respect to each other (*vibrational*) (infrared), (3) nuclei rotating about an axis (*rotational*) (infrared), and (4) electrons spinning about nuclei (*electronic*) (ultraviolet, visible). In the normal or ground state, the total energy possessed by a molecule is the sum of all these. If we add energy in the form of radiation, part of this will be

Table 2. Electromagnetic Spectrum, Approximate Ranges of Common Radiations

	ν 10^x Hz.	λ 10^x cm.
	$x = 0$	$x = 10$
		9
	2	8
Audible sound		7
	4	6
		5
AM broadcast	6	4
		3
FM broadcast		
	8	2
TV broadcast		
		1
Microwaves		
	10	0
Radar		−1
	12	−2
Infrared		−3
	14	−4
Visible		
		−5
Ultraviolet	16	−6
		−7
X-rays	18	−8
		−9
γ-rays	20	−10
	22	
Cosmic rays		

absorbed by the molecules, and if we can relate the energy absorbed to the energy administered, we get an *absorption spectrum* of the molecule in question.

To excite a molecule of a given structure requires a certain amount of energy which, if we supply it, will raise the ground state energy to a higher level, $E_0 \rightarrow E_1$.

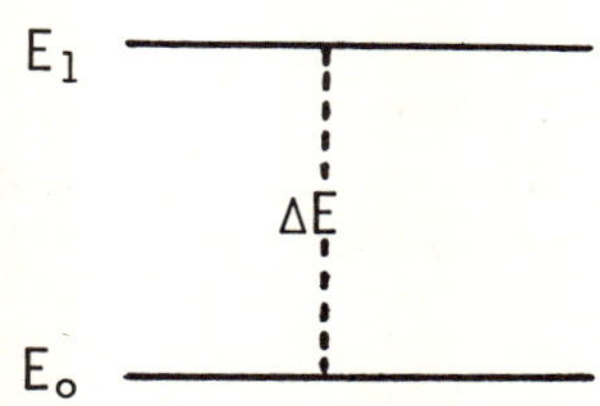

The amount of energy absorbed is the difference between the two levels and is proportional to the frequency of the radiation used.

Eq. 2 $$\Delta E = h\nu$$

h = Planck's constant, 6.6 = 10^{-27} erg sec.

If it were possible to excite only a single electronic state to produce a single transition $E_0 \rightarrow E_1$, we would expect absorption at a specific wavelength to produce a *line* as, for example, in *emission spectra*. But the molecules with which we are concerned can usually undergo several transitions, so we do not get a line but an *absorption band* with a maximum at λ where the line would be if there were one. Bands may be more or less sharply defined.

What happens to absorbed energy after the source of excitation is removed? The molecule, in relaxing from its excited state, gives up energy which may result in (1) heat (molecular collision) (infrared), (2) light (ultraviolet), (3) ionization (loss of electrons), (4) fragmentation of the molecule (dissociation into radicals), and (5) chemical reaction (photochemistry).

Not just any energy will excite a molecule. Remember that $\Delta E = h\nu$; a spectrum will result if the energy chosen is appropriate to the transition to be brought about.

VISIBLE SPECTROSCOPY

The *visible spectrum* is probably the most familiar to us all. White light is broken up by a prism or by rain drops to produce light of various colors, i.e., various wavelengths. We are also aware of colors such as those due to dyestuffs in cloth, paper, paint, etc. because dyes absorb all wavelengths but those reflected or transmitted which we see. Thus we see yellow because a dye absorbs blue. The wavelengths involved in visible light are measured in a number of ways. It is convenient to deal with this region of the spectrum in terms of wavelength rather than frequency, and the following expressions are used:

$$1\ \mu\ \text{(micron)} = 10^{-3}\ \text{mm.} = 10^{-4}\ \text{cm.}$$

$$1\ \text{m}\mu\ \text{(millimicron)} = 10^{-7}\ \text{cm.} = 1\ \text{nanometer (nm.)}$$

$$1\ \text{Å (Ångstrom unit)} = 10^{-8}\ \text{cm.}$$

Analytical procedures for some compounds may be based on direct measurement of the colors of their solutions, for example, $CuSO_4$ (blue) and Na_2CrO_4 (yellow), and colored organic compounds may be analyzed in this way. However, many other substances require the addition of a reagent which can yield a dye or a colored molecule for determination in the visible portion of the spectrum. We may refer to the visible portion of the spectrum from time to time, but other spectral regions which we will consider in the discussions which follow have greater importance. The visible spectrum includes the range of 400 to 700 nm.

ULTRAVIOLET SPECTROSCOPY

Ultraviolet absorption is an important characteristic of many organic drug molecules. The energies in this region of the spectrum are in the range of 5 to 10 e.v.; wavelengths are in the range of 200 to 400 nm. = 2000 to 4000 Å. What sort of excitation does such energy produce? Three classes of electrons can undergo transitions at these energy levels:

1. Electrons with *saturated bonds* (σ) are represented, for example, by the pairs of shared electrons in the paraffin hydrocarbons. They are relatively inert to added energy and ordinarily quite stable chemically. The energy required to disrupt these bonds, i.e., to move the electrons, is available only in the far ultraviolet. For this reason alkanes are often used as solvents for compounds to be measured in the normal ultraviolet (UV) spectral regions. We will not be additionally concerned with this class.

2. *Nonbonding electrons (n)* are those unshared electrons of hetero atoms such as N:, S:, O:, or halogen; they are the electrons which enter easily into complex formation (p. 39). They are less firmly bound than σ-electrons, but some still require a fair amount of energy

to bring about a transition $E_0 \rightarrow E_1$; for example, R—OH and R—O—R absorb only in the far ultraviolet. Thus ethanol can be used as a solvent for many UV determinations. In R—SH, R—S—S—R, R—I, or R—NH_2 there is some absorption in the near ultraviolet because the *n*-electrons are more weakly held and these bonds are somewhat weaker.

3. *Unsaturated bonds* (π), as the organic chemist knows, are weaker and more susceptible to chemical attack. Their electrons can undergo transitions at longer wavelengths (lower energy levels) than σ or *n* electrons. Tables of these bond types can be found in some of the more specialized texts on the subject, notably in J. R. Dyer's *Applications of Absorption Spectroscopy of Organic Compounds* (Prentice-Hall) or in R. M. Silverstein and G. C. Bassler's, *Spectrometric Identification of Organic Compounds* (John Wiley & Sons).

Most simple, single, or isolated double bonds absorb in the far ultraviolet; they require more energy for excitation than is available in the region we are attempting to study. There are, however, a few exceptions:

Compound	*nm.*
Acetaldehyde	290 weak
Acetone	279
Acetyl chloride	220
Acetamide	208–220
Nitromethane	271–274
Alkyl nitrite	218–220, 356 weak
Nitrosobutane	300 weak
	665 weak (visible, blue)

In benzenoid compounds, bonds are not isolated and the situation becomes more complex. Two bands are seen in simple benzene derivatives: 200 to 230 nm. moderate, 250 to 280 nm. weak. Similar tables for these are available in the references cited above.

Electronic groupings which absorb energy to produce color are called *chromophores*. Although we have indicated that this absorption may be weak, moderate, or strong, the intensity of the absorption may be quantitatively expressed by means of the *extinction coefficient* (ϵ) which, as we shall see, has significance in the analytical applications of the spectroscopic method. For the moment it is only necessary to recognize its existence and to note the effect produced by the introduction into a molecule of certain substituents which are capable of changing it. These substituents are called *auxochromes;* they change not only the position of the absorption maximum but the intensity of the absorption as well. An example of their effect can be seen as a result of their contribution of *n*-electrons to the π-electron system of the benzene nucleus:

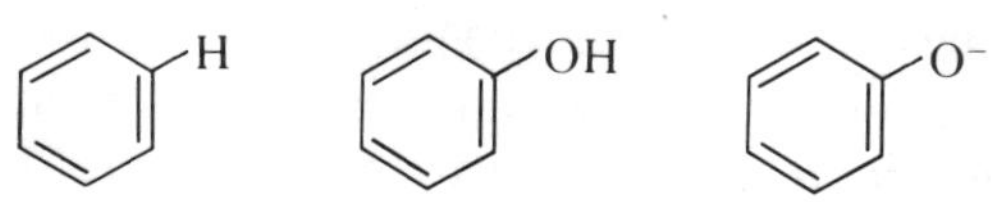

λ	203.5	254	210.5	270	235	287 nm.
ϵ	7400	204	6200	1450	9400	2600

Groups such as NH_2, SH, and some halogens do this. Slight effects are also noted from alkyl groups attached to simple unsaturated linkages:

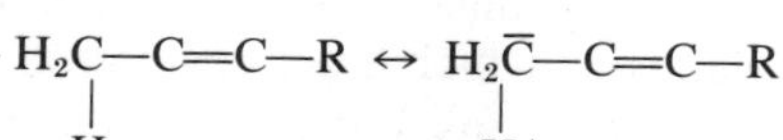

Multiple chromophores such as C═C—C—C═C (isolated) and —C═C—C═C— (conjugated) are a different matter as are conjugated carbonyl compounds, —C═C—C═O. Conjugation decreases the energy required to bring about electronic transitions. This is reflected in a shift of the absorption band 15 to 45 nm. toward longer wavelengths, the so-called *bathochromic shift*.

	nm.		
CH_3—CH═O	160	180	290 (weak)
CH_2═CH—CH═O		218	320 (weak)
CH_3—CO—CH_3	166	189	279 (weak)
CH_3—CH═CH—CO—CH_3		224	314 (weak)

By observation and experience, rules have been developed for the estimation of the effects of substitution on the ultraviolet spectra of various chromophores. These are known as *Woodward's rules* and are a basis on which the absorption maximum can be predicted for certain types of compounds. Base values are assigned to specific structures; the addition of chromophoric groups to these structures modifies the expected absorption in a predictable way. A brief summary of these rules and some examples of their application are given here.

1. Acyclic or cyclic nonfused conjugated dienes

—C═C—C═C— or 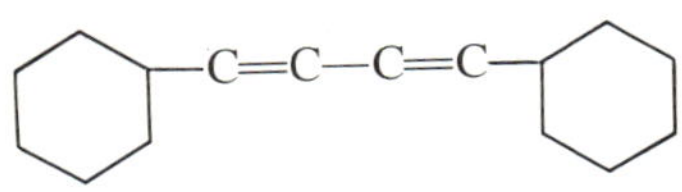

BASE = 217 nm.

for each alkyl substituent on the diene system	add	5 nm.
for each ring to which the diene is exocyclic	add	5 nm.
for each Cl or Br on the diene system	add	17 nm.

2. Cyclic fused rings — BASE = 217 nm.
   (a) heteroannular = diene system distributed between two rings

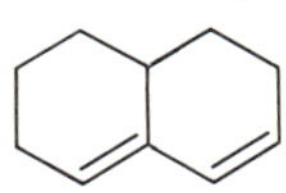

(b) homoannular = diene system in the same ring	add	36 nm.
In either (a) or (b):		
for each alkyl group on the diene system	add	5 nm.
for each ring to which —C═C— (d.b.) is exocyclic	add	5 nm.

3. α,β-unsaturated carbonyl compounds (aldehydes and ketones)

—C═C—C═O — BASE = 214 nm.

for each α-substituent (alkyl, alkoxy, acetoxy)	add	10 nm.
β-substituent	add	12 nm.
ring to which —C═C— is exocyclic	add	5 nm.
—C═C— + —C═O in a 5-membered ring	subtract	10 nm.
—C═C— in a 5-membered ring	add	5 nm.
α- or β-enolic OH	add	35 nm.

α-Cl	add	15 nm.
α-Br	add	23 nm.
extension of conjugation, per unit	add	30 nm.
δ- and γ-substituents on diene system	add	18 nm.

While these rules have applicability to a wide variety of compounds, they have their principal use in steroids and similar polynuclear compounds. A few examples will show how they work.

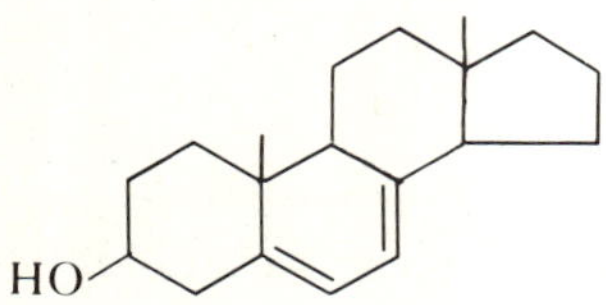

BASE =	217 nm.
homoannular diene	36 nm.
4 alkyl @ 5 each	20 nm.
2 rings, exocyclic d.b.	10 nm.
λ_{max} estimated	283 nm.
found	282 nm.

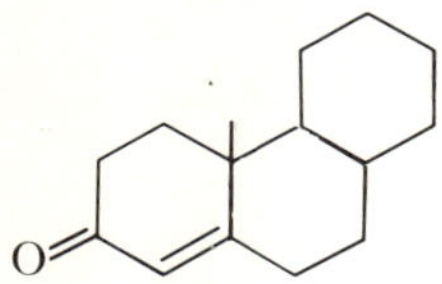

BASE =	214 nm.
2 β-alkyl groups @ 12	24 nm.
1 ring, exocyclic d.b.	5 nm.
λ_{max} estimated	243 nm.
found	241 nm.

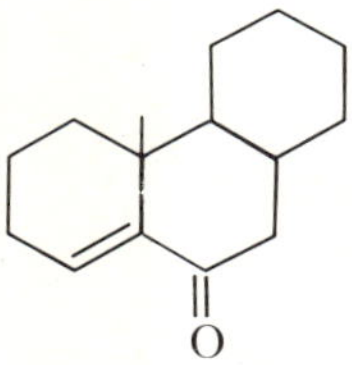

BASE =	214 nm.
1 β-alkyl	12 nm.
1 ring, exocyclic d.b.	5 nm.
1 α-alkyl	10 nm.
λ_{max} estimated	241 nm.
found	241 nm.

Thus, qualitatively, ultraviolet spectroscopy permits a number of things: (1) an overall view of the electron distribution in a molecule; (2) recognition of the probable presence of specific atomic groupings, e.g., conjugated carbonyl; and (3) estimation of the location of substituents by the degree of shift in absorption maxima. It permits also the quantitative estimation of substances which absorb in this wavelength region.

Two types of instruments are used: The single beam instrument consists of an H_2-lamp as a source of ultraviolet light, a rotatable prism for selection of wavelength, a slit to create a narrow beam of light, a cell for the sample (quartz, not glass), and a detector (photomultiplier tube). In use the instrument is calibrated at 100 percent transmittance (zero percent absorbance) with the solvent (blank) used in the determination so that the measured absorption is due only to the substance being studied. The double beam instrument differs from the single beam in that the chosen wavelengths are split to travel through the same length of solvent (blank) as the sample, for which the instrument automatically compensates. The rotating prism is coupled to a motor drive and the detector to a moving pen so that the absorption curve is drawn as it is produced.

Samples are usually run in solution; the solvent must be transparent to the wavelength chosen. The cells are usually of 1 cm. path length (sometimes 10 cm.). Concentrations are chosen so that absorption is within reasonable limits; 1 percent solutions are commonly used.

Given, then, the capability of producing excitation energy of a suitable magnitude and of recording the response by a given compound, it is possible to obtain an absorption spectrum for that compound in which the wavelength of maximum absorption will be characteristic for the compound or one very similar to it. If we can relate the degree of absorbance to concentration, we have a method for quantitative estimation.

For most absorbing substances, whether the absorbance lies in the ultraviolet or the visible range, the intensity of absorbance (or transmittance) is proportional to the concentration over some specified range. This is known as *Beer's law*. Usually very dilute or very intensely colored solutions depart from this rule. Without attempting to derive the relationships, we can say that

Eq. 3 $$\log I_o/I = abc$$

where I_o is the intensity of the incident light and I is the intensity of the transmitted light after passing through a layer of thickness (b) containing a substance in concentration (c); a is a constant. Other important expressions are:

where T = transmittance $$T = I/I_o$$

where A = absorbance $$A = \log[1/T]$$

Eq. 4 $$A = abc$$

A value for a is determined by measuring A with b and c known. If a remains constant over a range of c, the substance is said to obey Beer's law. You may see these relationships expressed in several ways.

$$A = \epsilon b c$$

where c is in moles/L. and ϵ is the molar absorptivity (liters/mole cm.), often called the extinction coefficient. *a* may also be expressed as $A^{1\%}_{cm}$, where c is in weight/volume units, e.g., grams/100 ml. An example of the use of the method follows:

Vitamin A has λ_{max} = 325 nm. with log ϵ = 4.7. An alcoholic solution (100 ml.) of a vitamin A preparation showed a measured transmittance of 60 percent in a 1 cm. cell. What is the concentration of the vitamin in the preparation? The molecular weight of vitamin A is 286.46.

$$\begin{aligned} A &= \log[1/T] \\ &= \log[1.0/0.6] \\ &= \log 1.666+ = 0.222 \end{aligned}$$

$A = \epsilon bc$, hence $c = A/\epsilon = 2.22 \times 10^{-1}/5 \times 10^4 = 0.444 \times 10^{-5}$ moles/L.; and $286.46 \times 4.44 \times 10^{-6}/10 = 1.27 \times 10^{-4}$ gm./100 ml.

FLUORESCENCE SPECTROSCOPY

We have already mentioned that electrons pushed into an excited state by the absorption of energy lose this energy in various ways in dropping back to their normal ground state. One of these ways was by the emission of radiant energy. The light emitted in this process is known as fluorescent light. *Fluorescence* exists as long as the excitation persists; it disappears when the excitation source is removed since often the time involved in the electrons dropping back to the ground state is only about 10^{-8} sec. If the process of dropping back takes a longer time, from 10^{-4} sec. to several days, the phenomenon is known as *phosphorescence*. You may have seen examples of this in displays of ores under ultraviolet light in a science museum. Both of these effects are included in the general term *luminescence*.

One might suppose that radiation emitted as fluorescence ought to be the same as the radiation absorbed. This is not the case; we find that the wavelength of the fluorescent light is nearly always longer than that of the excitation. The spectra ought to be mirror images of each other (see figure below) but this is not always observed. Many compounds absorb

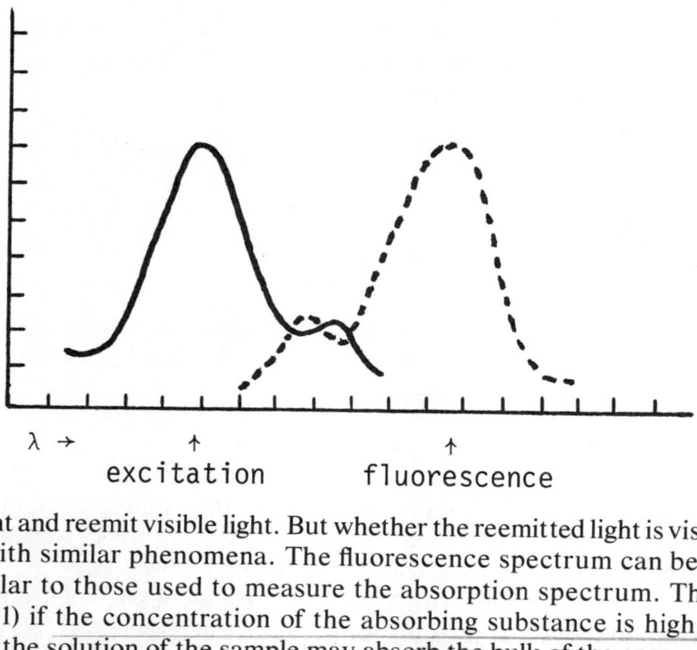

ultraviolet light and reemit visible light. But whether the reemitted light is visible or not, we are dealing with similar phenomena. The fluorescence spectrum can be measured by methods similar to those used to measure the absorption spectrum. There are a few differences: (1) if the concentration of the absorbing substance is high, the first few millimeters of the solution of the sample may absorb the bulk of the energy supplied, and the solution will fluoresce in an abnormal manner. Therefore concentrations used in fluorescence analysis are kept at very low levels. (2) Calculations are slightly different.

$$F = 2.3\, I_o \phi abc$$

where: F = fluorescence intensity ("absorbance")
I_o = incident radiation intensity
ϕ = quantum yield of fluorescence (varies from 0 to 1)
a, b, and c = their usual significance
$\phi = F/I_{absorbed}$.

In contrast to absorbance, fluorescence is proportional to the intensity of the incident light. Therefore, we can increase the sensitivity of the method by using low concentrations of substance and increasing I_o. This is done by using high-intensity mercury or xenon arc lamps. Since F is proportional to molar absorptivity (a), we use a wavelength for excitation close to or at λ_{max} for the compound to be analyzed. The instrument (see figure, p. 101) is also somewhat different than that used in ultraviolet spectroscopy.

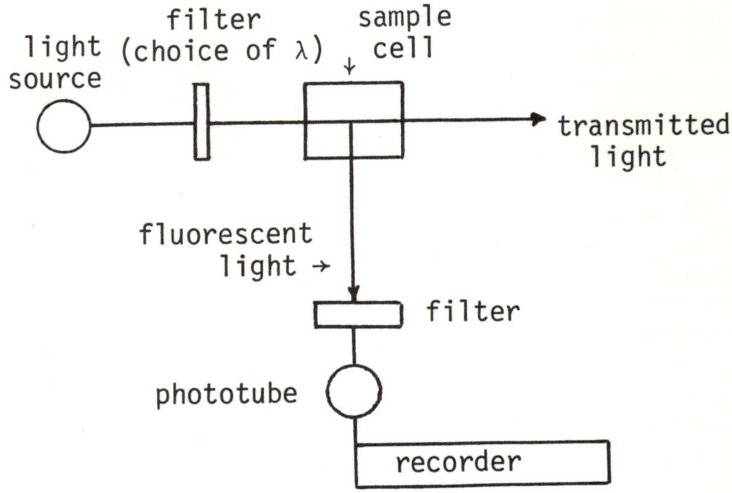

Fluorescence analysis has been applied to a number of drugs in drug abuse screening programs. Typical procedures may be found in an article by K. K. Kaistha.* LSD is a good example because of the very small amounts of the drug usually encountered when it is detected. After extraction of the drug from, for example, 5 ml. of appropriate biological fluid, an aliquot of the extract is shaken with HCl and allowed to stand for a few minutes. The fluorescence of the acid phase is determined at 445 nm. using 325 nm. as the wavelength of excitation. Metabolites of LSD are reported not to interfere in this determination.

THINGS TO REMEMBER

$$\nu = c/\lambda \qquad \Delta E = h\nu$$

$$A = \log [1/T] = \alpha bc = \epsilon bc$$

Woodward's Rules

Experiment 13. Spectrophotometric Assay of Sulfathiazole

> NOTE: The cuvettes (sample holders) for the spectrophotometer are to be handled with tissues. Clean the lower portion of the cuvettes before inserting them into the cell holder of the instrument, keeping this clean lower portion free of finger marks.

Standardization. Students may work in groups of four or five, pooling volumetric flasks used in making dilutions. If necessary, extra flasks will be supplied.

1. Weigh accurately 100 mg. of sulfathiazole which has been previously dried. Transfer it quantitatively to a 100 ml. beaker and dissolve it in about 40 ml. of 1 N HCl, stirring and heating if necessary. Cool and transfer the liquid quantitatively to a 100 ml. volumetric flask, dilute to volume with 1 N HCl and mix thoroughly. Transfer a 25.0 ml. aliquot to another 100 ml. volumetric flask, dilute to volume with the HCl solution, mix thoroughly, and label this "stock solution."
2. Fill a clean, dry buret with this stock solution. To each of four numbered volumetric

*Kaistha, K. K.: *Drug abuse screening programs: Detection procedures, development costs, street-sample analysis, and field tests.* J. Pharm. Sci. 61:655, 1972.

flasks (100 ml.) add 10, 14, 18, and 22 ml. of stock solution respectively. (The volumes need not be exactly 10.00, 14.00, etc., but they must be known accurately, i.e., 10.15, 14.20, etc.) Add 20 ml. of vanillin solution (graduated cylinder) to each flask, swirl to mix the contents, dilute to volume with HCl solution, and mix thoroughly.

3. Prepare a blank by dilution of 20 ml. of the vanillin solution with the 1 N HCl in a 100 ml. volumetric flask.

4. Check the spectrometer to insure that it is set at 390 nm., the wavelength to be used in this determination. Adjust it to read zero transmittance. To a cuvette add a suitable volume of the blank vanillin solution and place it carefully into the cell holder of the instrument. Adjust the spectrometer to read 100 percent transmittance.

5. Replace the blank with a cuvette containing the first sulfathiazole solution. Record the absorbance and the transmittance. Take five readings, inserting the blank occasionally to make sure that the instrument has not drifted from the original 100 percent transmittance setting. Repeat this with the other standard solutions, and report the mean values for A and percent T for each of the four solutions.

Determination. Now weigh accurately 100 mg. of your unknown and repeat step 1. If there is any solid present which does not dissolve, filter the solution directly into the volumetric flask using filter paper previously wet with 1 N HCl. After filtration, dilute to volume by passing the HCl solution through the paper to wash it thoroughly. Mix well and label this "unknown stock solution."

7. Using a buret, transfer 20.00 ± 0.20 ml. of this solution to a 100 ml. volumetric flask, add 20 ml. of the vanillin solution, dilute to volume with the HCl, and mix well.

8. Determine A and percent T for this solution as outlined in step 5. The determination of the unknown is to be done by the individual student.

9. Calculate the absorbance for the solutions used in the standardizations. Do they differ from those you recorded? If so, how do you account for the difference? Prepare a Beer's law plot from the calculated values. From the mean value for the absorbance of the unknown, refer to the graph and calculate the sulfathiazole content of your sample, reporting the result as percent purity.

Experiment 14. Spectrophotometric Determination of Ethyl Alcohol

Interest in the determination of ethanol for legal reasons has resulted in numerous accepted methods for its assay ranging from oxidation (p. 48) to gas chromatography, to an enzyme assay which is used here. The procedure uses the enzyme alcohol dehydrogenase which catalyzes the following reaction:

$$CH_3CH_2OH + NAD \xrightarrow{\text{enzyme}} CH_3\text{—}CHO + NADH$$

Under proper conditions, the amount of ethanol can be determined by measuring the optical density at 340 nm.; commercial kits containing necessary reagents are available for the purpose from, for example, Sigma, Calbiochem, or other suppliers. In the following experiment the Sigma kit was used.

Standardization. Students may work in groups of five.

1. Prepare a diluted ethanol standard by mixing 1.0 ml. of distilled water, 1.0 ml. of 6.25 percent trichloroacetic acid, and 0.5 ml. of ethanol, and cap the mixture until ready for use.

2. Into five NAD-ADH vials pipet the solutions indicated in the second and third columns below:

Vial no.	*Buffer (ml.)*	*Diluted Ethanol Standard (ml.)*	*Equivalent Percent Ethanol*
1	4.10	0.00	0.00
2	4.05	0.05	0.04
3	4.00	0.10	0.08
4	3.95	0.15	0.12
5	3.90	0.20	0.16

Allow the vials to stand capped at room temperature for approximately 30 min. Timing does not have to be accurate.

3. Transfer the contents of each vial to a spectrophotometer tube and read the optical density or percent transmittance at 340 nm. Tube 1 will serve as a blank.

4. Plot these values against ethanol concentration. The graph will not necessarily be a straight line, but it will pass through the origin.

Determination. In this portion of the experiment students work independently.

1. Into a centrifuge tube, pipet 2.0 ml. of 6.25 percent trichloroacetic acid followed by 0.5 ml. of your unknown ethanol sample. Seal the tube with a rubber stopper and mix by inverting a few times. Centrifuge this sample for 5 min.

2. Into each of two NAD-ADH vials pipet 4.0 ml. of pyrophosphate buffer, cap the vials, and invert them to dissolve contents.

3. Mark one vial "blank" and add to it 0.05 ml. of water and 0.05 ml. of 6.25 percent trichloroacetic acid. Mark the second vial "test" and add to it 0.1 ml. of the supernatant liquid from step 1.

4. Cap both vials. Mix by inversion and allow to stand at room temperature for about 30 min. Transfer the contents of each tube to a spectrophotometer tube, and read the optical density or percent transmittance at 340 nm. Use the blank to adjust the instrument.

5. Determine the percent concentration of ethanol in your sample by reference to the calibration graph.

PROBLEMS

1. Calculate the expected absorption maxima for the following compounds.

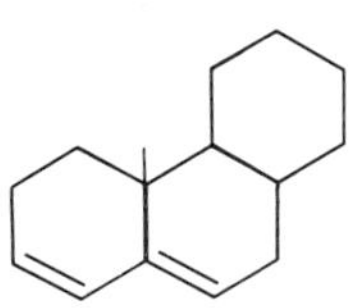
(a)

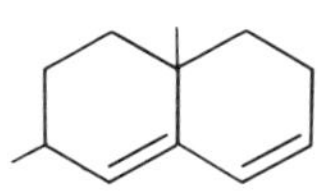
(b)

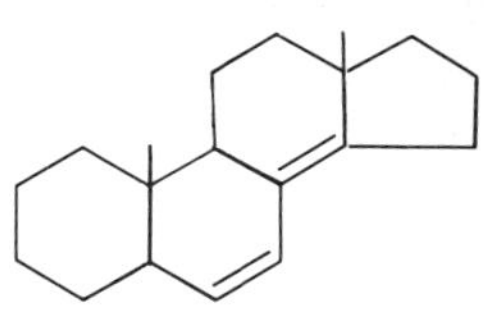
(c)

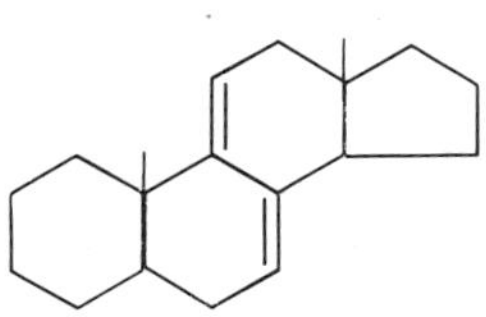
(d)

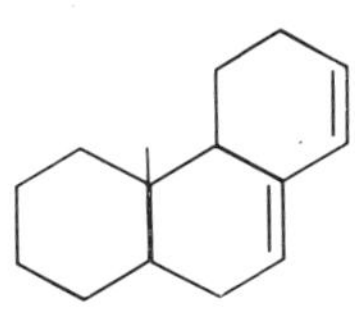
(e)

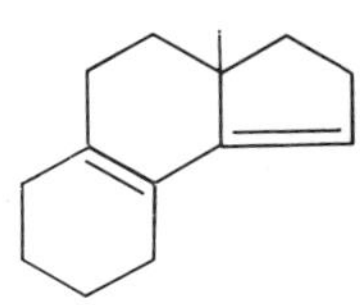
(f)

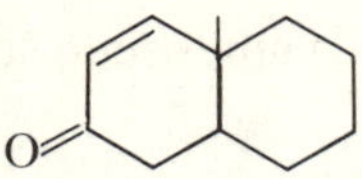

(g)

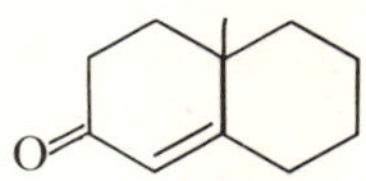

(h)

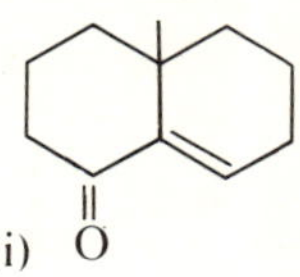

(i)

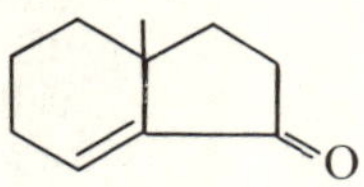

(j)

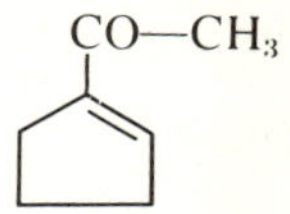

(k)

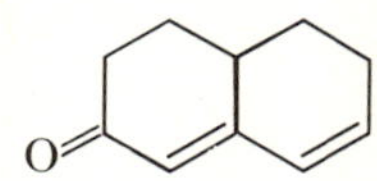

(l)

2. Triamcinolone, a synthetic corticosteroid, is represented by the following structure:

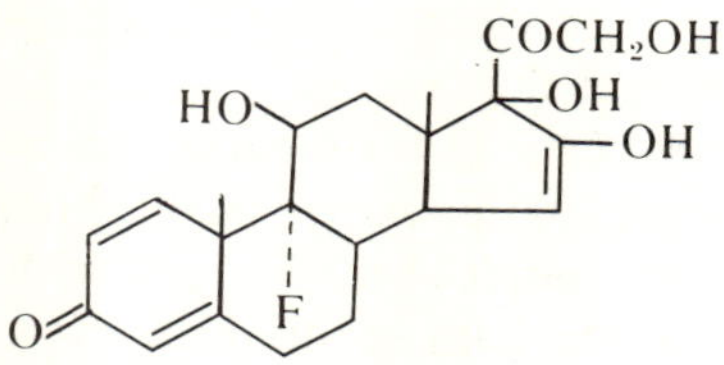

(a) A solution (0.0016 percent in ethanol) scanned between 210 and 340 nm. showed a *single* absorption band with ϵ = 15,900. At what wavelength was the maximum observed?

(b) The following specific rotations have been reported for the compound: +75° (c = 0.20 in acetone, t = 25°C.); +71° (c = 0.35 in acetone, t = 23°C.); +67.1 ± 1.9° (c = 0.5 in methanol, t = 22°C.); +70.5° (c = 1 in dimethylformamide, t = 21°C.). Give reasons for the apparent discrepancy in these results. Which value do you find most acceptable? Why?

(c) The specific rotation of the acetonide of triamcinolone, taken in a 2 dm. tube (c = 0.5 in dimethylformamide) was given as + 124°. What rotation was actually observed at the time of the determination?

3. Acetanilid has molar absorptivities of 10,000 in water at 240 nm. and 13,000 in benzene at 239 nm. A sample was dissolved in water and extracted once with benzene. The phases were separated and their ultraviolet absorptions were measured in a 1 cm. cell to give the following results: aqueous layer, 56.8 percent transmittance at 240 nm.; and benzene layer, 5.14 percent transmittance at 239 nm. Calculate the partition coefficient for acetanilid in the benzene-water system.

ANSWERS

1. (a) 237
   (b) 237
   (c) 247
   (d) 247
   (e) 237
   (f) 247
   (g) 226
   (h) 243

(i) 241
(j) 241
(k) 241
(l) 279
2. (a) 237 nm.
(c) 1.24°
3. 4.04

Chapter 12

Infrared Spectroscopy

The principles which we have discussed concerning the ultraviolet region are applicable to the other side of the visible spectrum, the infrared (IR). The wavelengths and frequencies involved are shown below.

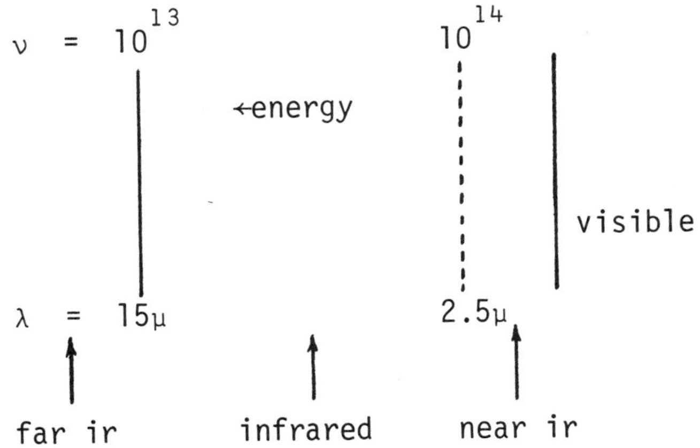

In this region we usually express the wavelengths in microns (μ) or in wave numbers (1/cm.); you will see both of these used in discussions of the subject. As in other absorptions, energy strikes molecules causing an excitation and consequent absorption of energy. In the infrared region, the relaxation, i.e., $E_1 \rightarrow E_0$, results in the production of heat rather than light as occurs in fluorescence. Another important difference between this spectral region and the ultraviolet is the fact that infrared frequencies excite not the electrons themselves but the molecules as a whole and, particularly, the bonds uniting the atoms to each other.

Individual atoms have nuclei with electrons spinning around them. They are attracted to each other by electrical forces of varying strengths (bonds). These bonds, while more or less stable, are not static; atoms are in some state of motion with respect to each other and can be conceived to vibrate in a number of ways. There are two fundamental types of vibration:

1. *Stretching*, the distance between the atoms increases or decreases along the bond axis.

symmetric asymmetric

Vibration is confined to the plane of the paper as these have been drawn.

2. *Bending,* the position of the atoms changes with respect to the bond axis. Perhaps it is easiest to understand these concepts by imagining the atoms as balls and the bonds joining them as springs. Bending vibrations may, but need not, be confined to a single plane.

A. In-plane bending:

scissoring rocking

A

B. Out-of-plane bending:

wagging twisting

B

When infrared radiation of the same frequency as these vibrations strikes a group of atoms, the amplitude of their vibrations increases, i.e., energy is absorbed. Theoretically this should occur at a specific frequency, but because rotational energies are superimposed on changes in vibrational energies simultaneously, we do not observe line spectra but bands of varying width. Because the vibrations we have discussed are examples of harmonic motion (springs!), we observe not only the fundamental bands but the overtones as well which are integral multiples of the fundamentals, as in music. Most of the deductions we can make using the infrared spectrum of a compound can be made using the fundamental bands; considerable experience may be necessary to recognize and interpret overtone bands.

The instrument used in this work usually has as its source of radiant energy a Nernst glowlamp, a filament of rare earth oxides heated to ~ 1500°C. The radiation is split into two beams, one for the sample and one for the solvent (blank). Wavelengths may be selected either by means of a prism or a grating. The more common instruments use a prism. Because glass and quartz are not sufficiently transparent to IR, the optics and cells used in the instrument must be made of other materials, chiefly inorganic halides:

NaCl	transparent from ~ 2 to 15.4μ
CaF_2	better for 2 to 7.7μ
KBr	useful from 9 to 35μ
CsBr	10 to 50μ; mostly for inorganics
AgCl	advantage: insoluble in water

Samples may be gas, liquid, or solid. We will not be concerned with gaseous samples. Liquids may be held in cells of ~0.1 mm. light path or in a liquid film between two halide plates. Solids may be handled in several ways:

1. Mulls may be prepared to suspend the solid in a hydrocarbon, e.g., Nujol or hexachloro-1,3-butadiene (good for the 3μ region). Nujol is more common but it has a spectrum of its own and because it is almost impossible to duplicate liquid films, a Nujol blank does not properly compensate. One must therefore discount the contribution of Nujol in the final interpretation of the spectrum.
2. Salt discs may be prepared by mixing sample and powdered KCl or KBr and compressing the mixture under high pressure to form a transparent disc. A blank should also be prepared. Sample to KBr ratio is of the order 2 to 4 mg./100 mg.
3. Films may be prepared by evaporation of a solution or cooling a melt. This is the least attractive method.
4. Solutions are often used for routine work. Concentrations range from 1 to 5 percent depending on the molecular weight of the compound under investigation, its chemical type, and cell thickness (usually 0.1 to 1 mm., 0.2 and 0.5 mm. are common). The instrument is adjusted so that the strongest band in the spectrum has a transmission of about 10 percent.

Solvents must be chosen carefully. Naturally the compound must be soluble, but water, alcohol, or hygroscopic solvents may not be used because of the sensitivity of the halide cells to these agents. Solvent absorption should be minimal in the spectral region under investigation; obviously the solvent should be incapable of reaction with the sample. Thus, commercial chloroform which contains 0.75 percent of ethanol as a preservative would not be suitable for an acid chloride since the ethyl ester would result. No single solvent is good for the entire 2 to 15μ range. For accurate work, two spectra may be taken using different solvents, e.g., CCl_4, CS_2, $CHCl_3$ (see Table 3).

The spectrum is recorded by the instrument on a piece of chart paper, the pen or the paper moving with change in wavelength, depending on the instrument. Paper shrinkage may make the recording of wavelength inexact so that calibration is necessary. Commonly a piece of polystyrene film is used which shows sharp bands at 6.24, 5.14, and 3.51μ; the 6.24μ band is more commonly used to provide a reference mark on the chart.

Interpretation of an infrared spectrum is not always a simple matter. Location of a characteristic absorption band (see Table 4, p. 110) as well as an estimation of its relative intensity expressed as *s* (strong), *m* (medium), *w* (weak), or *v* (variable) is necessary. It should be clear from previous discussions that vibrations for all similar kinds of atom pairs, e.g., $-C=O$, will not be identical but will be influenced by the environments of these

Table 3. Regions of the Infrared Obscured by Solvents and Other Media

Material	*Regions Obscured*
Carbon tetrachloride	840–700 (11.90–14.30)
Carbon disulfide	1600–1400 (6.25–7.15)
Chloroform	3000 (3.33)
	1200 (8.33)
	840–700 (11.90–14.30)
Nujol	3000–2900 (3.33–3.45)
	1470–1440 (6.80–6.45)
	1385–1365 (7.27–7.33)
Potassium Bromide*	3500–3300 (2.86–3.03)

*If the pellet contains water. Since the water content may vary appreciably, the interpretation of this region of a spectrum determined in a potassium bromide pellet is *always* subject to error.

atoms, Hence, we cannot say that an absorption band will fall in a characteristically reproducible place in the spectrum but rather that it will fall within a given area or range. Several variables modify any selected absorption band including: (1) position, (2) shape, (3) effect of the change in medium and (4) intensity. For these reasons, interpretation becomes an important part of any IR determination.

To summarize, we might say that:

1. IR spectra can give a wealth of information about the nature and structure of molecules.
2. Many interpretations must be made with caution and after considerable experience.
3. The method is not a substitute for traditional chemical methods but it can be very helpful in suggesting structures of unknown compounds or in confirming structures arrived at by other means.
4. The lack of absorption is often most diagnostic; it rules out the existence of certain functional groups.
5. On the other hand, the identity of an IR spectrum with that of a known compound, coupled with, for example, melting point (m.p.), mixed m.p. and other data such as the optical rotation, is a virtual guarantee of identity.

To aid you in the interpretation of IR spectra in the laboratory experiments which will require it and to illustrate the principles we have discussed above, characteristic IR absorption frequencies are given in Table 4. Similar and much more extensive tables can be found in specialized texts such as those cited in Chapter 11.

Table 4. Representative Infrared Absorption Frequencies

3μ region (3600–2500 cm.$^{-1}$)		Stretching vibrations of H bonded to C, O, N. Care should be exercised in the interpretation of very weak bands as these may be overtones (2ν) of strong bands in the 6μ region.
2.78 – 3.13 (3600–3200)	OH	3600 (sharp), unassociated OH; 3400 (broad), associated OH. Both bands are frequently present in alcohol spectra. With strongly associated OH (COOH or enolized β-dicarbonyl compounds) the band is very broad (~500 cm.$^{-1}$) with its center at 2900–3000.
2.94–3.13 (3400–3200)	NH	3400 (sharp), unassociated NH; 3200 (broad), associated NH; an NH_2 group usually appears as a doublet (separation ~50 cm.$^{-1}$); the NH of a secondary amine is often very weak.

Table 4. Representative Infrared Absorption Frequencies—*continued*

3.00 (3300) 3.25 (3080) 3.28 (3050)	CH of —C≡CH of —CH=CH_2 of aromatic	The complete absence of absorption in this region indicates the absence of H bonded to C=C or C≡C and usually indicates the lack of unsaturation in the molecule. Since this absorption may be very weak in large molecules, some care should be exercised in the interpretation of this region.
3.36–3.45 (2980–2900)	of —CH_2—CH_2—	As in the previous entry, complete absence of absorption here indicates absence of aliphatic CH bonds.
3.45–3.64 (2900–2750)	of —CH=O	Either one or two bands may be found in this region for a single aldehyde function in the molecule.
4–5μ region (2300–2000 cm.$^{-1}$)		Stretching vibrations of triple bonds.
4.45–4.50 (2250–2225)	—C≡N	Nitrile absorption is often difficult to interpret in this region.
4.65–4.76 (2150–2100)	C≡C	This band will be either very weak or absent if the acetylene is approximately symmetrical.
6μ region (1900–1550 cm.$^{-1}$)		*Usually* stretching vibrations of C=C, C=O and C=N.
5.85 (1710)	C=O of aldehyde or ketone	This value refers to the carbonyl absorption frequency of a nonconjugated aldehyde or ketone with no electronegative groups near the carbonyl group. Since this frequency is altered in a predictable way by structural alterations, the following generalizations may be made:
	—C=C—C=O —C=C—CO—C=C—	1. *Effect of conjugation.* Conjugation of the carbonyl group with an aromatic ring or a C—C double or triple bond lowers the frequency by ~30 cm.$^{-1}$. If the carbonyl group is part of a cross-conjugated system (unsaturation on either side of the carbonyl group), the frequency is lowered by ~50 cm.$^{-1}$. Thus an aryl alkyl ketone or an alkyl vinyl ketone would absorb at about 1680 whereas a diaryl or divinyl ketone would absorb at about 1660.
		2. *Effect of ring size.* Carbonyl groups in 6-membered and larger rings exhibit approximately the same absorption as acyclic ketones. The C=O absorption frequency is raised ~35 cm.$^{-1}$ per atom decrease in ring size. A cyclopentanone absorbs ~1745. The effects of conjugation and ring size are additive, e.g., a 2-cyclopentanone absorbs at ~1710.
	—C—CO—C— (X on the first C)	3. *Effect of electronegative atoms.* An electronegative atom, especially oxygen or halogen, bonded to the α-carbon atom of an aldehyde or ketone may raise the position of the carbonyl absorption frequency by ~20 cm.$^{-1}$. Since this effect is dependent on molecular conformation, such compounds may exhibit normal absorption, absorption at higher frequencies, or both.
5.75 (1740)	—CO—OR	This band is subject to all of the structural effects described above. Thus, a conjugated ester absorbs at ~1710 cm.$^{-1}$ and a γ-lactone at ~1780.
6.02 (1660)	—CO—NH_2	This band is lowered in frequency by ~20 cm.$^{-1}$ by conjugation and raised by 45 cm.$^{-1}$ per unit decrease in ring size.
5.56 (1800)	—CO—Cl	As in the case of ketones, the frequency is lowered by conjugation.

Table 4. Representative Infrared Absorption Frequencies—*continued*

5.52 and 5.68 (1800 and 1760)	—CO—O—CO—	Both bands are present. Each is altered by ring size and conjugation to approximately the same extent noted for aldehydes and ketones.
5.88 (1700)	—CO—OH	This absorption frequency is lowered by conjugation as noted for aldehydes and ketones.
6.06–6.25 (1650–1600)	—C═C— of an olefin	1650, usually weak, indicates unconjugated olefin; 1610, medium to strong, conjugated olefin. The absorption bands at these frequencies are raised by ring strain but to a lesser extent than noted for the carbonyl functions.
6.10 (1640)	—C═N stretch	This band is usually weak.
6.25–15μ region (1600–600 cm.$^{-1}$)		This is the so-called "fingerprint region" usually associated with single band stretching vibrations, with bending and other more complex molecular vibrations. The positions of the absorption frequencies in this region are much less reliable than those discussed above. In addition, many bands interfere with one another and as a result only a portion of the bands in this region can be interpreted with reliability; interpretation is often questionable.
6.25 (1600)	—NH_2 bending	This band, in conjunction with the bands in the 3μ region, is often used to characterize primary amines and unsubstituted amides.
6.50 (1540)	—NH bending	This band, also in conjunction with bands in the 3μ region, is often used to characterize secondary amines and monosubstituted amides. In the case of secondary amines this band, like the band in the 3μ region, may be very weak.
6.58 and 7.41 (1520 and 1350)	—NO_2 coupled stretching	This pair of bands is usually very intense.
7.09 (1465)	—CH_2 bending of methylene next to carbonyl	
6.90 and 7.28 (1450 and 1375)	—CH_3	The band of lower frequency (1375) is usually used to characterize a methyl group. If two methyl groups are bonded to one C-atom, a characteristic doublet (1385 and 1365) will be present.
10.25 (970)	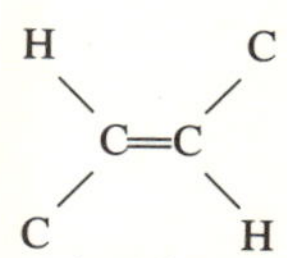 bending	This strong band is present in the spectra of *trans*-1,2-disubstituted olefins.
10.25 and 11.00 (975 and 910)	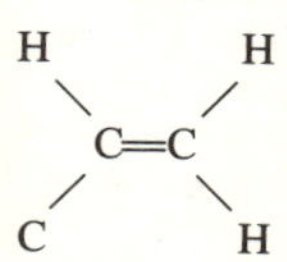	The lower frequency band of these two strong bands is used to characterize a terminal vinyl group.
11.20	—C—CH_2—	This strong band, used to characterize a methylene

Table 4. Representative Infrared Absorption Frequencies—*continued*

(890)	—C—H bend	group, may be raised by 20-80 cm.$^{-1}$ if the methylene group is bonded to an electronegative group or atom.
14.30 (700)	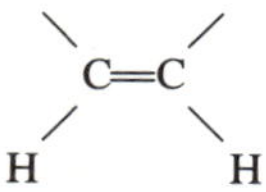	This band, attributable to a *cis*-1,2-disubstituted olefin, is unreliable because it is frequently obscured by solvent absorption or other bands.

The following bands are indicative of substitution patterns in benzenoid compounds. Since they may be obscured by solvent absorption or other bands, they are of use only when obtained from spectra made with the KBr disc and then care should be exercised in their interpretation.

13.30 and 14.50 (750 and 690)	CH bending of a monosubstituted benzene.
13.30 (750)	CH bending of an *ortho*-disubstituted benzene.
12.80 and 14.30 (780 and 700)	CH bending of a *meta*-disubstituted benzene.
12.10 (825)	CH bending of a *para*-disubstituted benzene.

As an example of how we might apply the knowledge we have gained thus far to a specific problem, let us consider a sample of mint oil which might have been tentatively identified by means of its index of refraction (p. 85). Chemical examination of this oil resulted in the isolation of a compound, $C_{10}H_{16}O$, which showed $[a]_D = +21°$, absorption maxima at 253 and 366 nm. (log $\epsilon = 3.911, 1.929$), and prominent infrared bands at the following wavelengths: 3.35, 5.95, 6.90, 7.30, 7.80, and 8.30μ. These data might cause us to reason:

1. The UV absorption suggests unsaturation;
2. The empirical formula suggests the possibility of an α,β-unsaturated carbonyl compound (see p. 97);
3. IR data confirm this with absorption at 5.95μ;
4. Aliphatic C—H (3.35μ) and the probability of a methyl group (6.90/7.30μ) are also indicated.

Reference to suitable literature (e.g., *Terpenes,* Vol. II of *Handbook of Naturally Occurring Compounds* by T. K. Devon and A. I. Scott, Academic Press, 1972) suggests several structures which might meet these criteria.

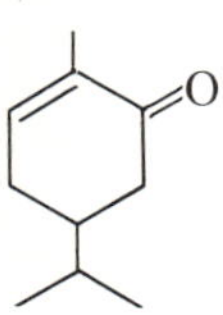

I
d-carvotacetone

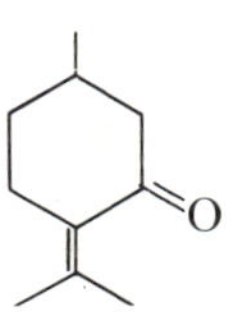

II
d-pulegone

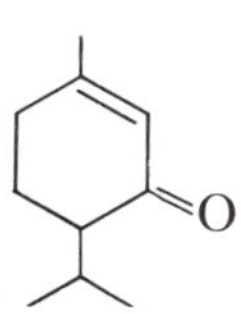

III
d-piperitone

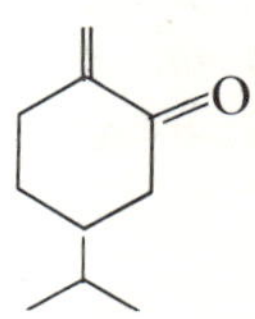

IV
santolineneone

Simple calculations of the anticipated absorption maxima by Woodward's rules (p. 97) predict that I should absorb at ~236 nm., II at 253 nm., III at 238 nm., and IV at 229 nm. Further, the $[a]_D$ for I, II, and III are given as 60, 28, and 62° respectively. The substance in question is therefore II; although $[\alpha]$ for IV is not recorded, the absorption maximum eliminates this possibility from serious consideration.

Experiment 15. Assignment of a Structure by Infrared Spectroscopy

Your instructor may wish to assign a simple unknown organic compound for which you are to obtain the spectrum and interpret it with reference to its major functional groups. Carry out one of the following procedures with his assistance.

1. If your unknown is a liquid, put a drop between the halide plates to create a "liquid film" and obtain a spectrum for this form.

2. If your unknown is a solid two procedures are available (a specific assignment will be made at the time of the experiment).

   (a) Weigh out 4 mg. of your unknown drug and add it to the shaker tube provided. Add 100 mg. of powdered potassium bromide. Stopper the tube and mix the powders intimately by shaking for a few seconds on the apparatus provided. Now, using the pellet press, compress this mixture to a small tablet. Use it to obtain a spectrum of the compound.

   (b) Weigh out about 5 mg. of your unknown. Grind it to a very fine dispersion in a drop of mulling agent (Nujol will be provided). Place the dispersion between the halide plates and obtain a spectrum of the compound.

If for some reason (low concentration, too dense a film, non-transparent KBr disc, etc.) your spectrum is not suitable for proper interpretation, consult your instructor about rerunning it.

Finally, interpret the spectrum in terms of the major absorption bands present, and on the basis of these interpretations, identify your "unknown."

PROBLEMS

1. A nonbasic compound, C_8H_9NO, gave an IR spectrum showing the following major absorption bands: 3.30, 5.92, 6.25, 6.58, 6.95, 7.30, and 14.50μ (3030, 1689, 1600, 1520, 1439, 1370, and 690 cm.$^{-1}$). Interpret these data in terms of a plausible structure for the compound.
2. To obtain an infrared spectrum of a substance suspected to be aspirin a student dissolved 5.0 mg. in 1.5 ml. of freshly prepared anhydrous ethanol and transferred a portion of this to a polished quartz sample cell of 1.0 cm. thickness. After calibration of the spectrometer using the 6.24μ band of polystyrene, the spectrum was taken. The result was unsatisfactory. Why?
3. List the major absorption peaks to be expected in the IR spectrum of prednisolone.

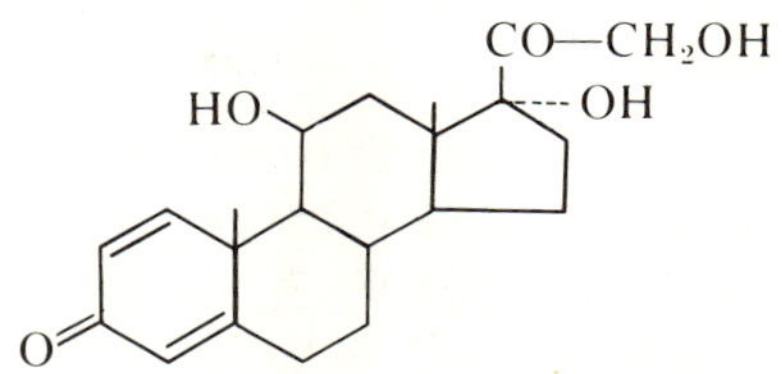

4. Interpret the spectrum below in terms of a compound with molecular formula $C_4H_8O_2$.

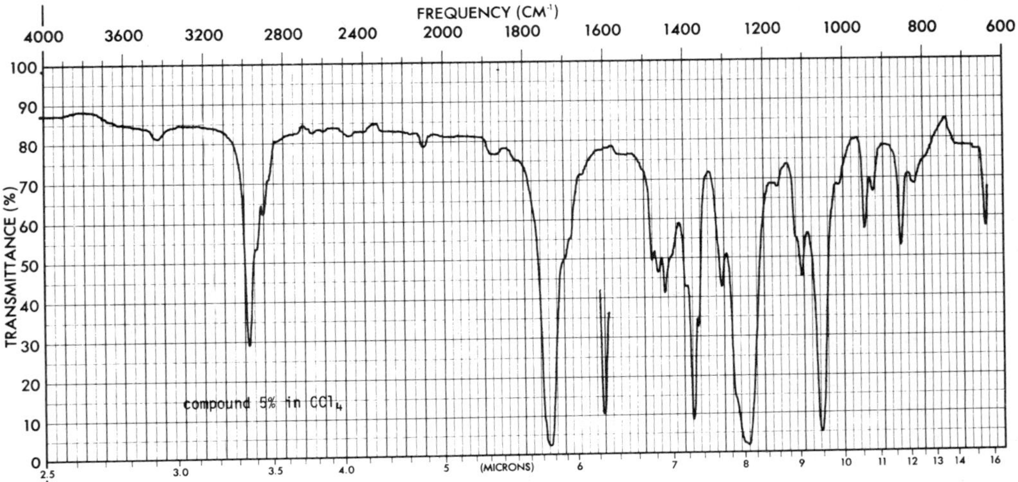

5. The compound which gave the spectrum below had a formula C_3H_7NO. What is its structure?

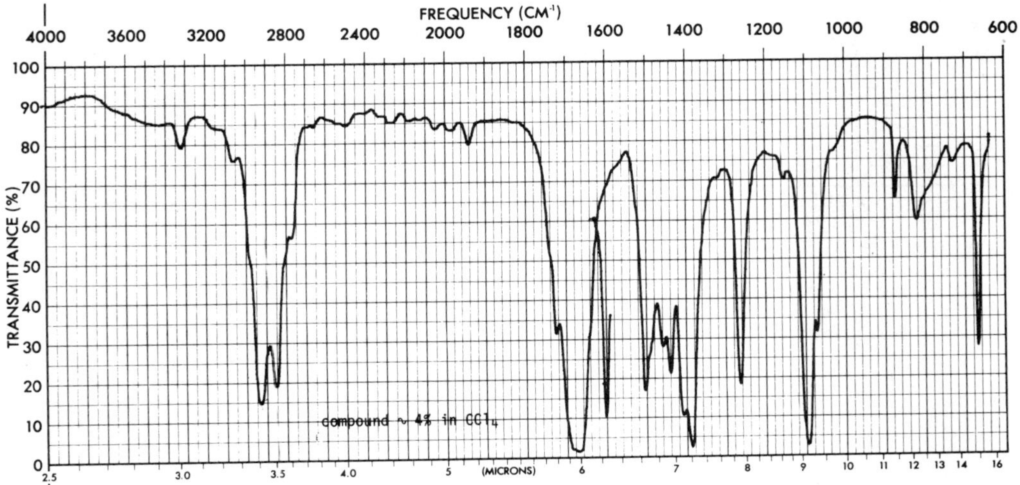

6. Interpret the spectrum below in terms of $C_4H_8O_2$.

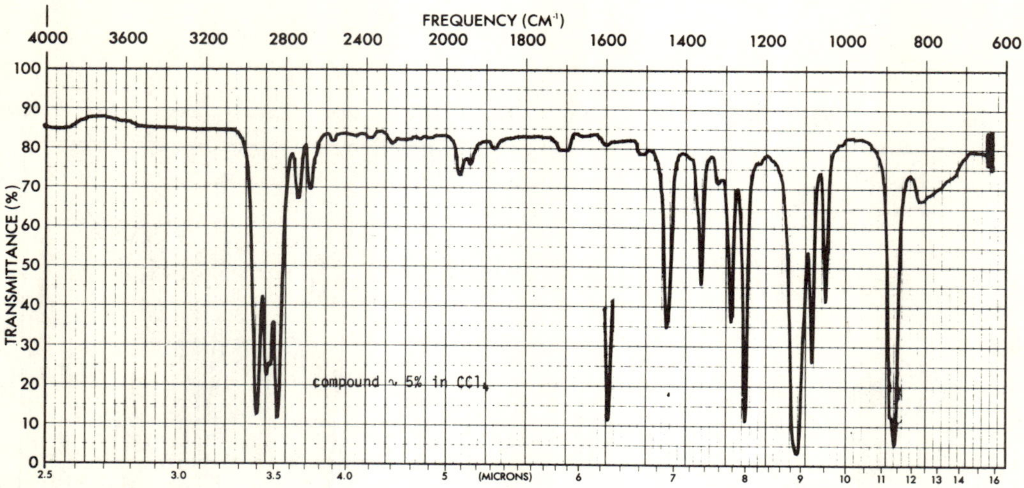

7. The compound which gave the spectrum below had a formula C_8H_{10}. Suggest a reasonable structure.

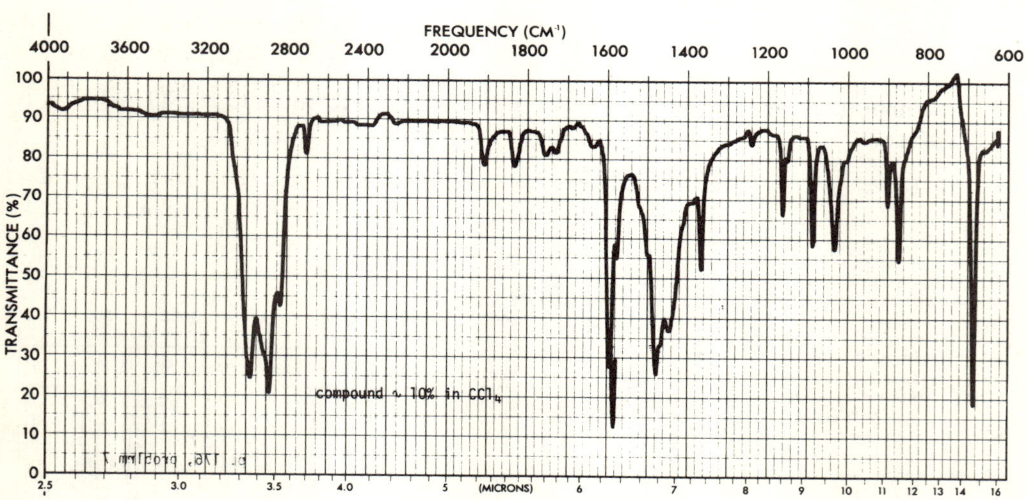

Chapter 13

Nuclear Magnetic Resonance Spectroscopy

We have seen that an ultraviolet spectrum gives something of an overall picture of a molecule, particularly of its electronic distribution. The infrared spectrum focuses on certain details of its structure, i.e., the nature of the functional groups. The nuclear magnetic resonance (NMR) spectrum gives us a look at even more specific features of the structure which, in combination with other data, make the method a valuable tool in the identification of organic compounds.

Nuclear magnetic resonance spectroscopy is based on principles that are somewhat different from those previously discussed. Recall that, in the classical picture of an atom, electrons spin around the nucleus in orbits like the planets around the sun. The nucleus, itself, is also considered to spin and, in certain atoms, the spinning nucleus develops a magnetic moment, that is, it acts like a small bar magnet (see figure below). This behavior of the hydrogen nucleus, the proton, will be our immediate concern. If a proton is placed in a magnetic field, its magnetic moment can align itself *with* that of the field or *against* it. It is more stable if it is aligned with it and has a tendency to stay that way. But, if we supply sufficient magnetic energy, we can flip it out of alignment and can measure the amount of energy necessary to do so.

This amount of energy depends on the strength of the magnetic field in which the proton is trapped. Perhaps the simplest analogy we might make is with a compass, the needle of which aligns itself north-south in the earth's magnetic field. If we supply energy in the form of a strong magnet near the compass case, or if you like, by a tap of the finger, the needle will flip out of its alignment and return when the energy is removed.

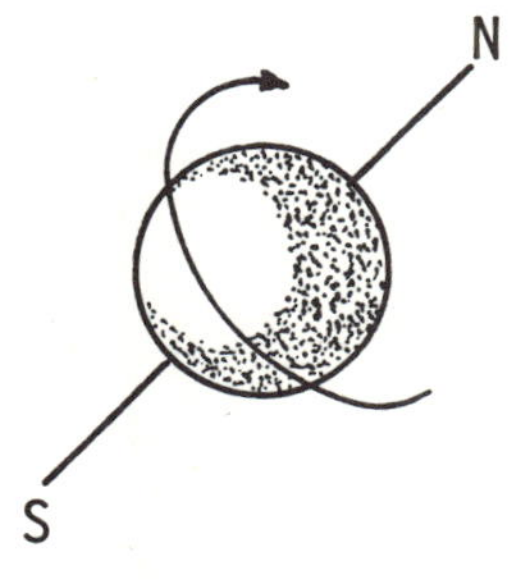

The relationship between the energy supplied and the magnetic field in which the proton is captured is given as follows:

$$\nu = \frac{\gamma H_0}{2\pi}$$

where ν = frequency (cps)
H_0 = magnetic field strength (gauss)
γ = "gyrometric ratio," a constant for a particular nucleus (26,750 for hydrogen).
There are, then, two ways to create the energy change necessary to flip a proton out of an established magnetic alignment:

1. Keep the magnetic field (H_0) constant and vary the frequency (ν) just as we did in the other spectral methods, i.e., "hit" the protons with radiation of different frequency (or wavelength, since $\nu = c/\lambda$), and observe the point at which absorption takes place.
2. Keep the frequency constant and vary the magnetic field. In practice, it is more convenient to do this. At some point in the field strength continuum, the energy required to flip the proton out of alignment is obtained, and a signal corresponding to absorption of energy will be received.

At first glance, this would seem to be simple. But not all protons are the same; they will give different signals depending on their environments (electron densities at the protons themselves; the groups to which they are attached). Thus, while the *effective field strength* may be the same for all protons, for any given proton it will depend on the environment of that proton which will then require a slightly different *applied field strength* in order to absorb energy.

The radiation frequency used in NMR spectroscopy is in the radio range (60 to 100 MHz.) which is of lower energy (lower frequency, longer wavelength) than the range for IR. It is, in fact, just beyond the FM broadcast band and in the TV frequency range. The instrument produces a constant radiofrequency, a variable magnetic field, and includes a detector for picking up signals representing absorption of energy. With it we can "look at" protons in a way which permits drawing a number of conclusions.

1. The *number* of signals tells us the number of *kinds* of protons in the molecule, all protons with the same environments giving the same absorptions.
2. The *position* of the signals (the location of the peaks) with reference to a standard tells us something about that proton environment.
3. The *intensity* of the signals tells us how many of each kind of proton there are—the higher the peak (more precisely, the greater the peak area), the greater the number.
4. The *splitting* of a peak into two or more peaks tells us something about the environment of that proton with respect to its neighboring protons.

Now let's apply these concepts to some simple examples:

Kinds of Protons

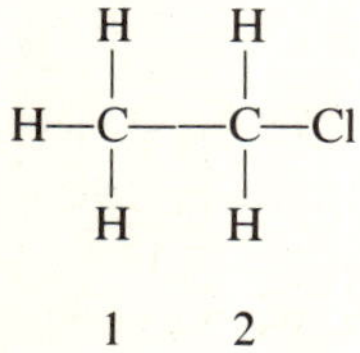

1 2

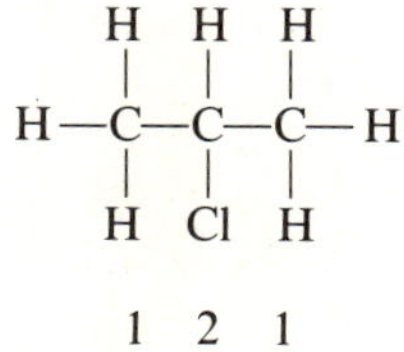

1 2 1

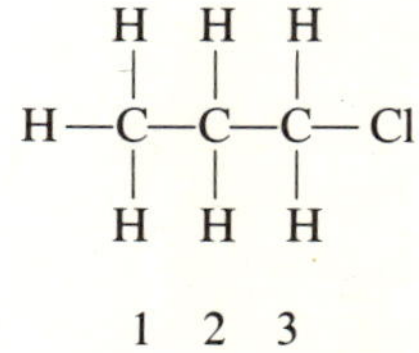

1 2 3

2 kinds	2 kinds	3 kinds
2 signals	2 signals	3 signals

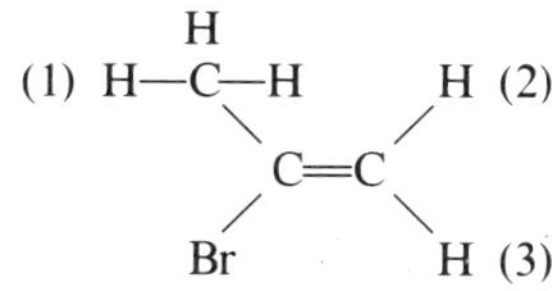

3 kinds

3 signals

Peak Position

The position of absorption—the location of signal peaks—tells us something about the environment of the protons present. For example, if we didn't already know the structures of the molecules above, how could we discover them by NMR? To answer this we must understand a few more basic principles:

1. Atoms have planetary electrons as well as nuclear protons.

2. If a molecule is placed in a magnetic field, not only are the protons influenced as we have seen but the electrons are caused to circulate as well. In doing so, they generate magnetic fields of their own (charge in motion = magnetism), *induced* magnetic fields.

(a) If the electrons circulate about the proton itself, the magnetic field thus generated is aligned so as to *oppose* the applied field. Hence, the applied field *felt* by that proton is less and the proton is said to be *shielded.*

(b) If the electrons circulate about a neighboring nucleus, the magnetic field generated can either (depending upon location of the proton): (1) *oppose* the field of the proton (shielding) or (2) *reinforce* the field of the proton (deshielding).

Thus, a shielded proton requires a higher applied field strength and a deshielded proton requires a lower applied field strength than a naked proton to provide the *effective* field strength for absorption. As a result, the shielded proton will absorb further up field ($\uparrow H_o$) than "normal;" the deshielded proton will absorb further downfield ($\downarrow H_o$).

These shifts are called *chemical shifts* and are expressed in parts per million (p.p.m.) of the total applied magnetic field, i.e., fractions of it. Actually, these shifts are shifts from the normal value of a naked proton, but for convenience, a *reference standard,* tetramethylsilane (Me_4Si), is used. Shielding of the protons in Me_4Si is much higher than in other organic molecules so that most signals appear downfield from those of Me_4Si, the proton absorption of which is taken as a reference point. Either of two scales is used to measure these shifts:

$$\tau \text{ with } Me_4Si = 10.0\text{; 10 to 0, downward}$$

$$\delta \text{ with } Me_4Si = 0.0\text{; 0 to 10, upward}$$

Often in texts or publications both are given ($\tau = 10 - \delta$). For an extensive list of chemical shifts for typical proton environments, the text of Dyer or Silverstein and Bassler (see p. 96) may be consulted. A somewhat abbreviated table is given at the end of this chapter.

The spectrum of toluene, C_7H_8 is reproduced below. Two signals are observed, i.e., two

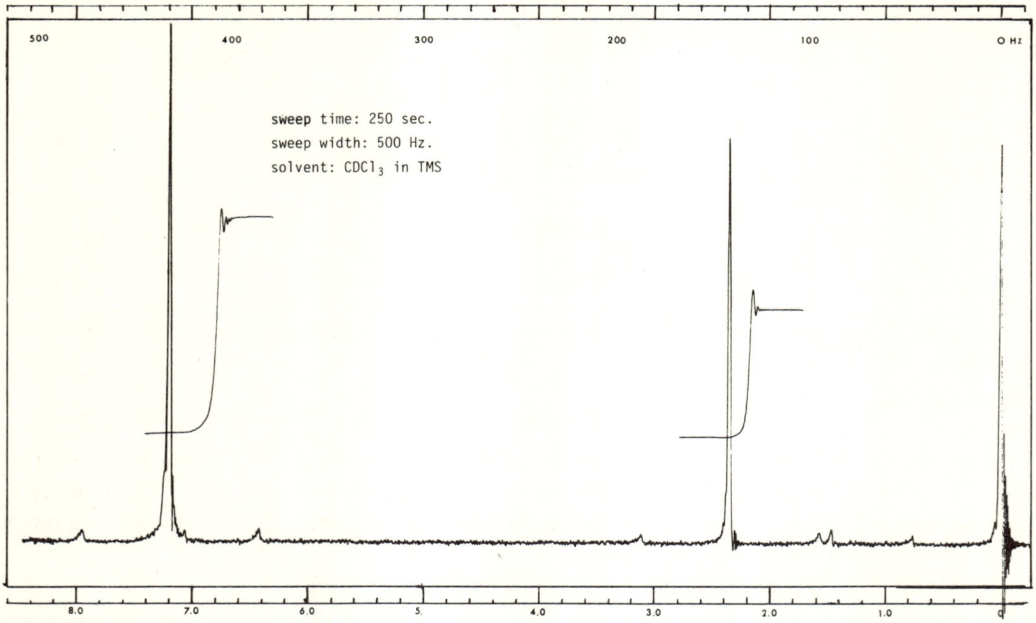

kinds of protons are present. These signals are at δ = 2.3 (τ = 7.7) and δ = 7.2 (τ = 2.8) p.p.m. corresponding to benzylic protons C_6H_5—$C\underline{H}_2$— (δ = 2 to 2.3 p.p.m.) and aromatic protons (δ = 6 to 8.5 p.p.m.), respectively. We can however, extract additional information from this spectrum.

Number of Protons

The number of protons is reflected in the area of the peak, i.e., the relative intensity of the signal. That is, the area under a signal peak is proportional to the number of protons giving that signal. This is reasonable because if a given kind of proton requires a given amount of energy to flip it in a magnetic field, *n* such protons will require $n\Delta E$.

If the curves in NMR spectroscopy were broad, such as the bands in UV or some absorption peaks of IR, we could arrive at a measure of the area under the curve by counting squares on the chart (graph) paper. However, this is difficult to do with the sharp peaks often seen in NMR spectra, so the instrument includes an electronic integrator to do this by tracing a curve in which step height is proportional to area.

If we study the spectrum of toluene in more detail, we see that the integrated peak height at δ = 2.3 p.p.m. corresponds to 5.2 units, while that at δ = 7.2 p.p.m. corresponds to 8.5 units. This represents a ratio of 1:1.7 or 3:5. There are, therefore, 3 "benzylic" protons and 5 aromatic protons in the molecule and we can write the structure of toluene as

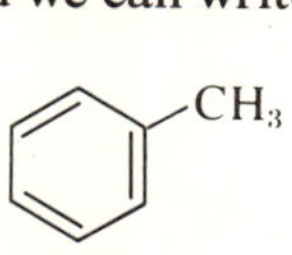

To take another example: a compound, C_7H_8O, gives a spectrum with proton peaks at δ = 3.65, 4.45, and 7.2 p.p.m. and peak heights in the ratio of 1.5:3:7 = 1:2:5. These correspond to:

δ	*Kind*	*Number*
3.65	R—O<u>H</u>	1
4.45	—C<u>H</u>$_2$—O—	2
7.2	Aromatic	5

The compound in question is thus described as benzyl alcohol:

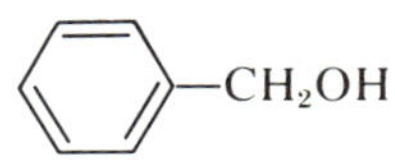

Suppose, as a final example, a compound of formula $C_{11}H_{16}$ revealed the following spectral data:

δ	*Assignment*	*Number*
7.15	aromatic	5
2.5	benzylic	2
0.9	methyl	9

The only compound which will fit these data has the indicated structure:

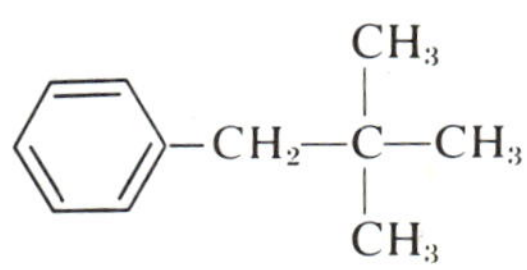

Signal Splitting

If we now apply these principles to some other types of compounds, we recognize apparent discrepancies in our knowledge. Consider, for example, the simple compound, dibromoethane:

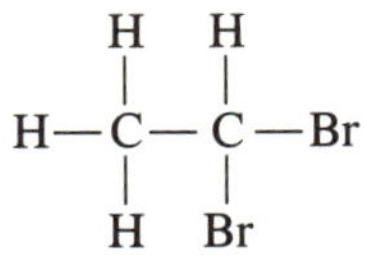

I

We can see two kinds of protons in the molecule, yet if we examine its spectrum, we count what appear to be six peaks!

What we have *not* done up to now is consider the effect produced on a given proton by other protons in its immediate environment.

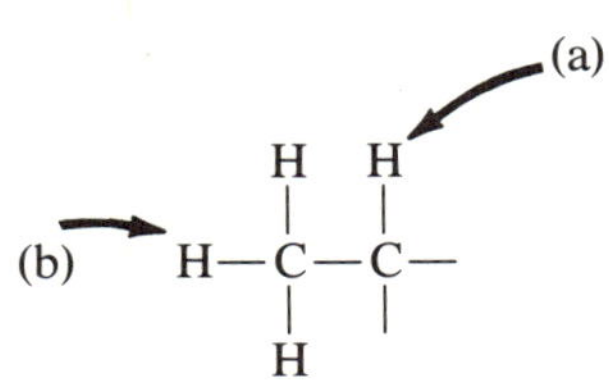

II

At any given instant, the spin of proton a may be aligned with the magnetic field thus slightly increasing the spin of b or, equally probably, against it, thus slightly decreasing it. The signal for the b protons (which are equivalent) becomes split into *two* peaks (doublet). By the same token, the signal for proton (a) will be split by the protons (b) to give *four* peaks. For II, then, the two signals are observed as a doublet and a quartet, rather than as two single spikes which might have been expected. This is called *spin-spin coupling* which produces multiplets whenever neighboring protons exert sufficient influence.

Generally, *a set of n equivalent protons will split an NMR signal into* n *+ 1 peaks.*

We may be able to make this clearer with a few examples.

III 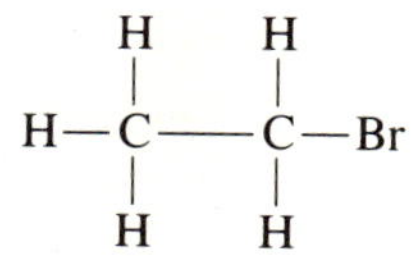

Thus in I above we can expect two peaks (two kinds of protons) split into a quartet and a doublet. For III, which also has two kinds of protons, we can expect the spectrum to show these two peaks split into a quartet and a triplet. Chemical shifts (v.s. Me_4Si) are consistent with the deshielding effect of halogens; protons on a C-atom containing a greater number of halogens will occur more downfield. The distance between peaks of split signals, e.g., a triplet, remains constant (J, expressed in cycles per second) for a given structural relationship between the coupled spins of the protons. Table 6 contains some common splitting patterns.

Finally, let's apply these rules to a few simple compounds.

Formula : C_3H_7Br

δ	*Splitting*	*Integration*	*Ratio*	*Structure*
0.9–1.2	triplet	11	3	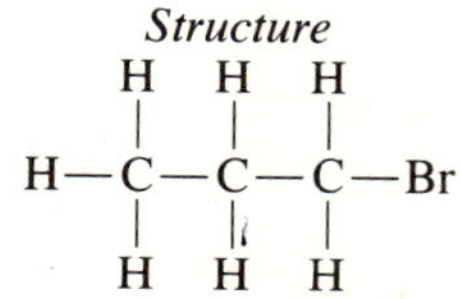
1.6–2.2	sextuplet	7.5	2	
3.4–3.5	triplet	7.0	2	

Formula : C_2H_6O

δ	*Splitting*	*Integration*	*Ratio*	*Structure*
5.3	singlet	5	1	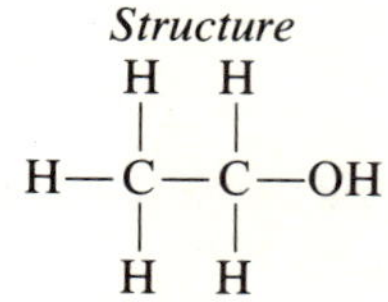
3.4–3.8	quartet	11	2	
1.1–1.4	triplet	15	3	

Formula : C_3H_8O

δ	*Splitting*	*Integration*	*Ratio*	*Structure*
1.1–1.4	doublet	29	6	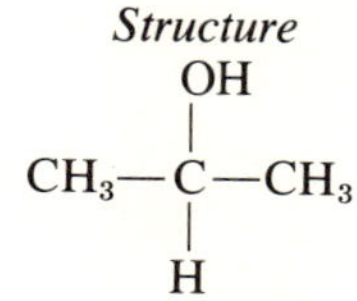
3.2	singlet	5	1	
3.7–4.1	septet	5	1	

Some of the common chemical shift values which will help interpret NMR spectra are given in Table 5; some of the common splitting patterns are listed in Table 6.

Table 5. Some Common Chemical Shift Values

Region (δ)	*Functional Groups*
0–1	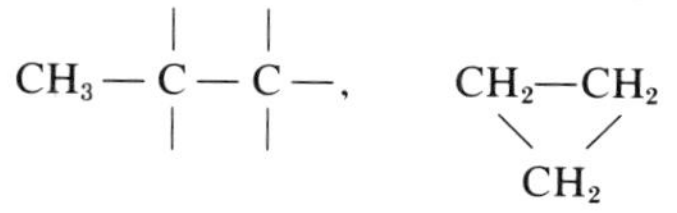
1–2	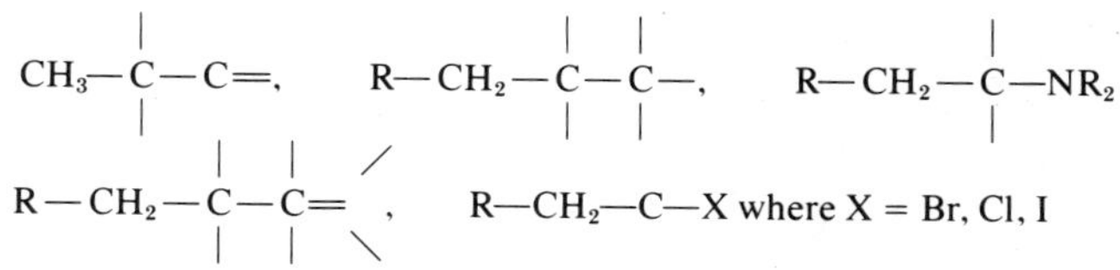 R—CH_2—C—X where X = Br, Cl, I
2–3	R—CH_2—CO—R where R = OH, NR_2, OR′; HC≡CH, R—CH_2CO—CH_2—R, R—CH_2—SH (↑ at CH_2); R—CH_2—NR_2, R—CH_2—C_6H_5 (↑ at CH_2)
3–4	HC≡C—C_6H_5 (↑ at H), R—CH_2—X where X = Br, Cl, I; R—CH_2—OR′ where R′ = H or alkyl (↑ at CH_2)
4–5	R—CH_2—O—CO—R, R—CH_2—F, 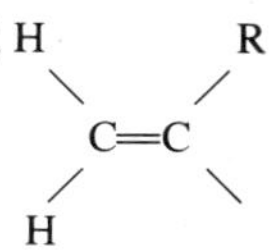
5–6	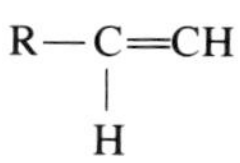
6–7	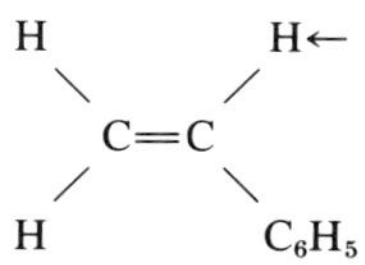
7–8	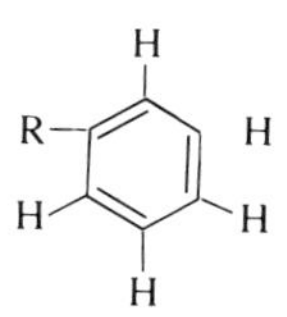 where R = alkyl, halogen, carbonyl
8–9	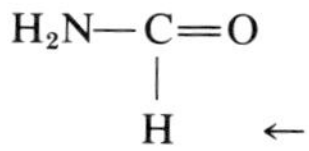
9–10	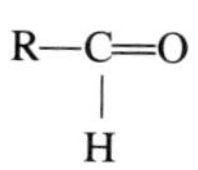 where R = alkyl
10–12	R—COOH
2–10	—OH concentration dependent
3–8	—NH_2 concentration dependent

Table 6. Some Common Splitting Patterns

Structure	*Protons*	*Splitting Pattern*	*Centered* δ *(p.p.m.)*
CH$_3$—CH$_2$—X, X = halogen	—CH$_2$— CH$_3$—	quartet triplet	3.0 1.8
X—CH$_2$CH$_2$CH$_2$—X, X = halogen	—CH$_2$—X	triplet	3.5
	—C—CH$_2$—C—	quintet	2.0
R—CO—OCH$_3$	CH$_3$—O—	singlet	4.2
R—CO—CH$_3$	CH$_3$—CO—	singlet	2.1
H$_a$ CO—R C=C H$_b$ CH$_3$	—CH$_3$ H$_a$ H$_b$	singlet singlet singlet	1.9 5.5 6.1
HC≡C—CH$_3$	—CH$_3$ HC≡	singlet singlet	1.8 1.8
CH$_3$—CH(Cl)—COOH	—CH$_3$ —CH(Cl)— —OH	doublet quartet singlet	1.7 4.5 11.2
CH$_3$O—CH$_2$—CN	—CH$_3$ —CH$_2$—	singlet singlet	3.5 4.2
CH$_3$—CO—CH(CH$_3$)(CH$_3$)	—CH—CH$_3$← CH$_3$—CO— —CH	doublet singlet septet	1.4 2.1 2.4
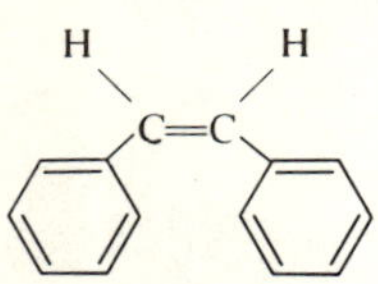	H—C=C—H 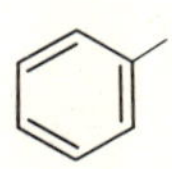	singlet singlet	6.5 7.2
H—CO—N(CH$_3$)(CH$_3$)	—N(CH$_3$)(CH$_3$) H—CO—	two peaks singlet	2.90, 3.0 8.0
H—CO—CH$_3$	—CH$_3$ H—CO—	doublet quartet	2.2 9.8

Table 6. Some Common Splitting Patterns—*continued*

Structure	*Protons*	*Splitting Pattern*	*Centered δ(p.p.m.)*
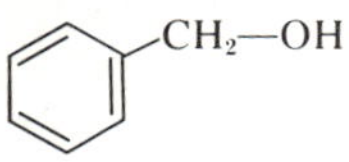	$—CH_2—$	singlet	2.4
	—OH	singlet	2–10
	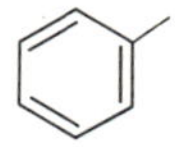	singlet	7.3
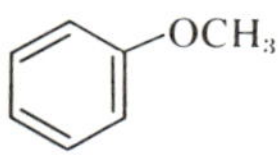	$—CH_3$	singlet	3.8
	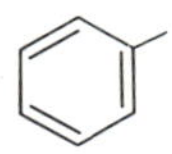	multiplet	6.8–7.5
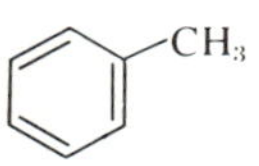	$—CH_3$	singlet	2.3
	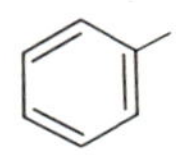	singlet	7.2
$CH_3—COOH$	$—CH_3$	singlet	2.1
	—OH	singlet	11.4

Example. An example of the application of NMR spectroscopy to a common analytical problem is the assay of APC tablets as described by D. P. Hollis.* Using a sweep width of 250 Hz., a setting on the instrument which determines the length of the chart span, the constituents of APC show sharp peaks and the δ-values indicated below in parentheses due to the protons to which they are assigned.

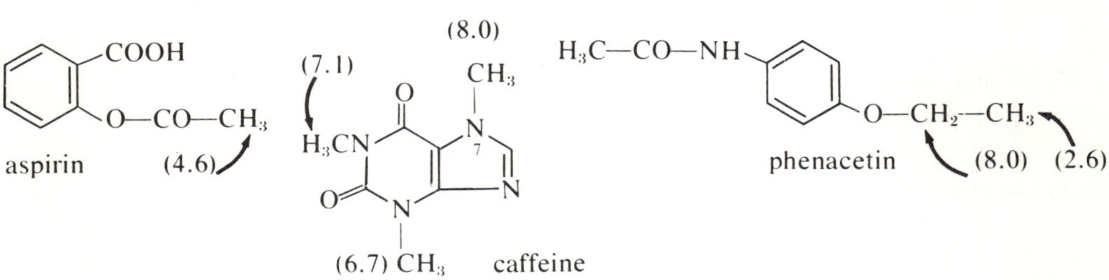

The three protons of the methyl group in aspirin represent one molecule of that substance. Measurement of both the 6.7 and 7.1 p.p.m. peaks gives six protons representing one molecule of caffeine. The methylene quartet of phenacetin at 8.0 p.p.m. is complicated by the N_7-methyl group of caffeine which absorbs at that point also. Thus, integration of the area under that multiplet represents two protons for each phenacetin molecule and three

*Hollis, D. P.: *Quantitative analysis of aspirin, phenacetin, and caffeine mixtures by nuclear magnetic resonance spectrometry.* Anal. Chem. 32:1682, 1963.

for each caffeine molecule. Since the number of caffeine molecules can be measured independently at the 6.7 and 7.1 peaks, the integration at 8.0 can be corrected for phenacetin by subtracting one-half of the 6.7 and 7.1 areas. Correcting all ratios to give molecular equivalents, the molar ratios of each of the ingredients are given by the following equation:

$$\text{Aspirin : caffeine : phenacetin} = I_a : [1/2\, I_c] : 3/2[I_p - 1/2\, I_c]$$

where I_a is the integration at 4.6 p.p.m., I_c is the integration at 6.7 and 7.1, and I_p the integration at 8.0 The *relative* concentrations can be calculated by including the molecular weights:

$$C_a : C_c : C_p = I_a(180) : 1/2\, I_c(194) : 3/2[I_p - 1/2\, I_c]\ (184).$$

The *absolute* concentrations can be calculated by comparison with a standard. A sample containing 500 mg. of caffeine in 5 ml. of solvent is examined under the same conditions as the unknown. The integration at 6.7 and 7.1 is recorded. The concentration of caffeine in the unknown (C_c) in milligrams per 5 ml. is proportional to the integrated areas for the reference sample and the unknown sample:

$$C_c = I_c \times C_{ref}/I_{ref}$$

The concentration of aspirin (C_a) and phenacetin (C_p) can then be determined by the following relationships:

1. $C_a/180\, I_a = C_c/(194)\, 1/2\, I_c$
2. $C_a = C_c I_a(180)/(194)\, 1/2\, I_c$
3. $C_p/(184) 3/2[I_p - 1/2\, I_c] = C_c/(194)\, 1/2\, I_c$
4. $C_p = [C_c \times 3/2[I_p - 1/2\, I_c]\ (184)/(194)\, 1/2\, I_c$

At the discretion of your instructor, and depending on the availability of time and of the instrument, you may have an opportunity to do the following experiment.

Experiment 16. Quantitative Analysis of APC by NMR spectroscopy.

NOTE: *Do not use the instrument unless the laboratory instructor is present.*

1. Weigh and powder 5 APC tablets in a small mortar and pestle.
2. Transfer 600 mg. of the powder, accurately weighed, into a 5 ml. centrifuge tube, add exactly 5.0 ml. of spectral grade chloroform and dissolve the powder as completely as possible.
3. After the powder has dissolved completely, transfer a small portion of the solution to an NMR tube.
4. Adjust the instrument using a tube of pure deuterated chloroform containing TMS.
5. Set the instrument for a 250 Hz. sweep width and 250 sec. sweep time (the time it will take the instrument to scan the chart); place your sample into the instrument and run your spectrum.
6. When the spectrum is complete, integrate the peaks which appeared between 10 and 2 p.p.m.

7. Place 500 mg. of a standard sample of caffeine into a centrifuge tube, add 5.0 ml. (pipet) of spectral grade chloroform and repeat steps 3 to 6.

8. Make the calculations discussed in the preceding portion of the text.

PROBLEMS

1. Indicate the major features of the IR and NMR spectra of the following:

(a)

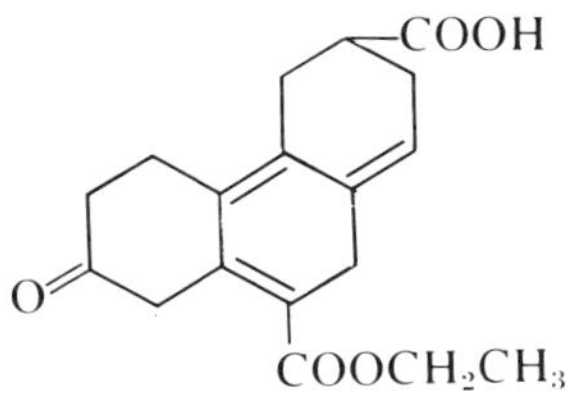

(b)

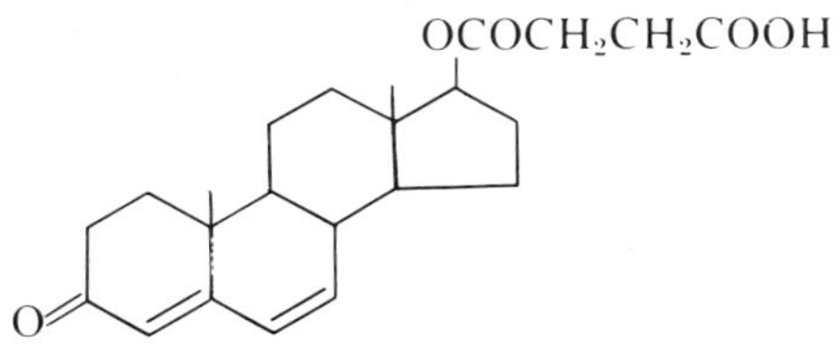

(c)

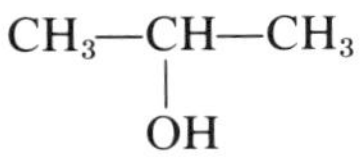

(d)

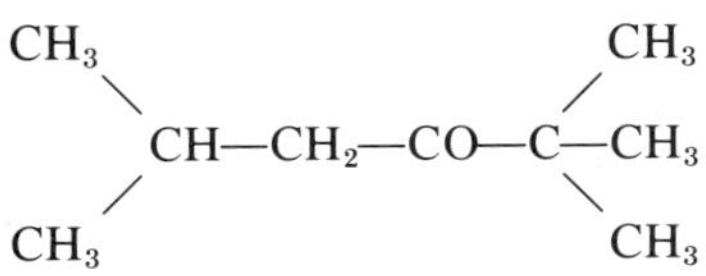

(e)

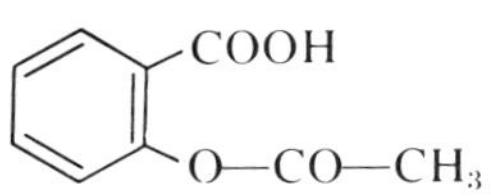

(g)

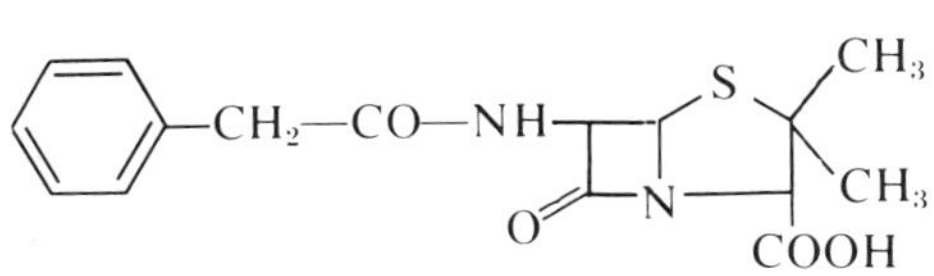

(f)

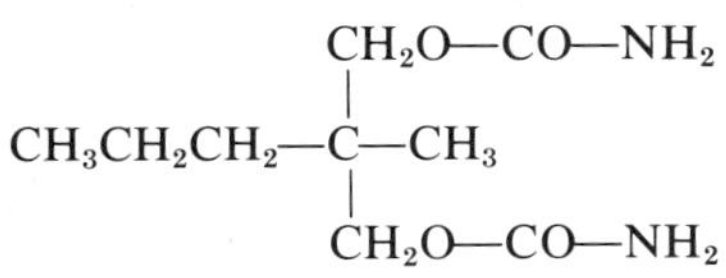

2. Interpret the spectra of the following compounds and suggest their structures. Compare the IR spectra of the same compounds in Problems 4 through 7 on p. 115–116.

(a)

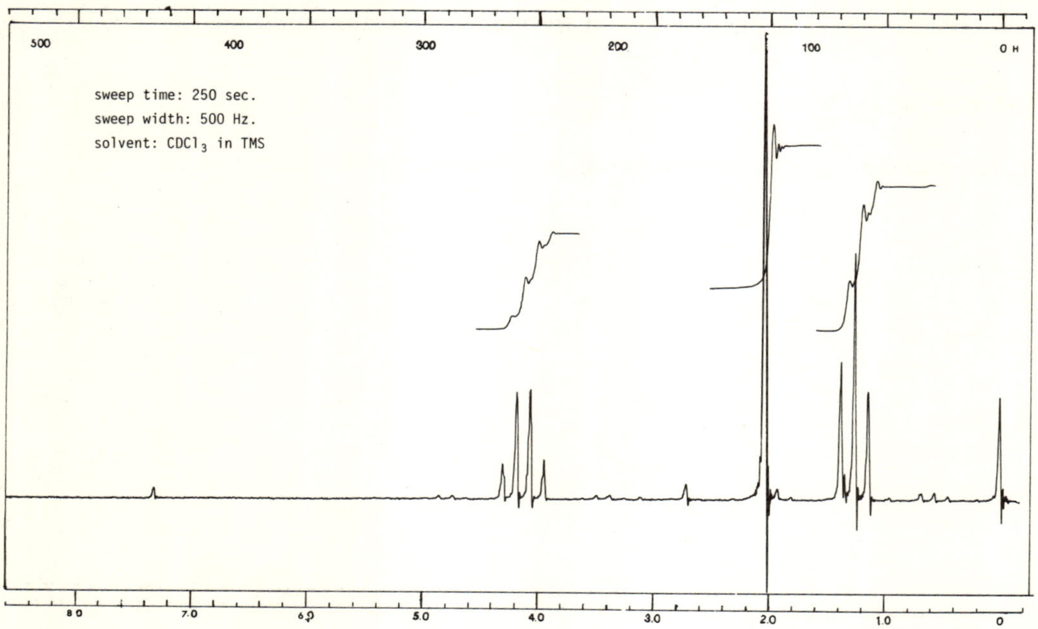
500
400
300
200
100
0 H
sweep time: 250 sec.
sweep width: 500 Hz.
solvent: CDCl3 in TMS
8.0
7.0
6.0
5.0
4.0
3.0
2.0
1.0
0

(b).

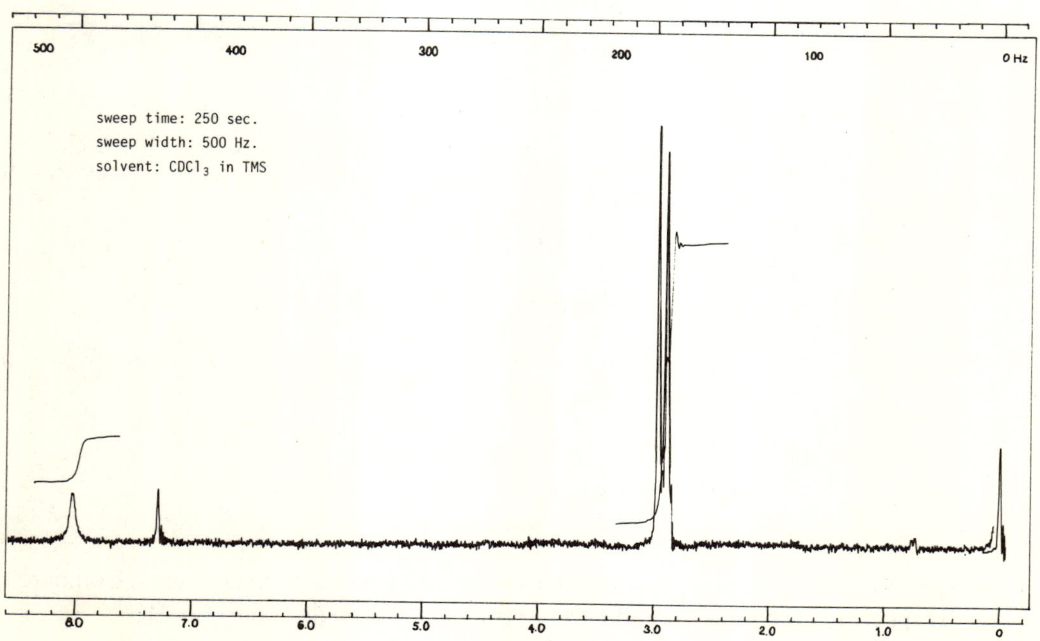
500
400
300
200
100
0 Hz
sweep time: 250 sec.
sweep width: 500 Hz.
solvent: CDCl3 in TMS
8.0
7.0
6.0
5.0
4.0
3.0
2.0
1.0
0

(c)

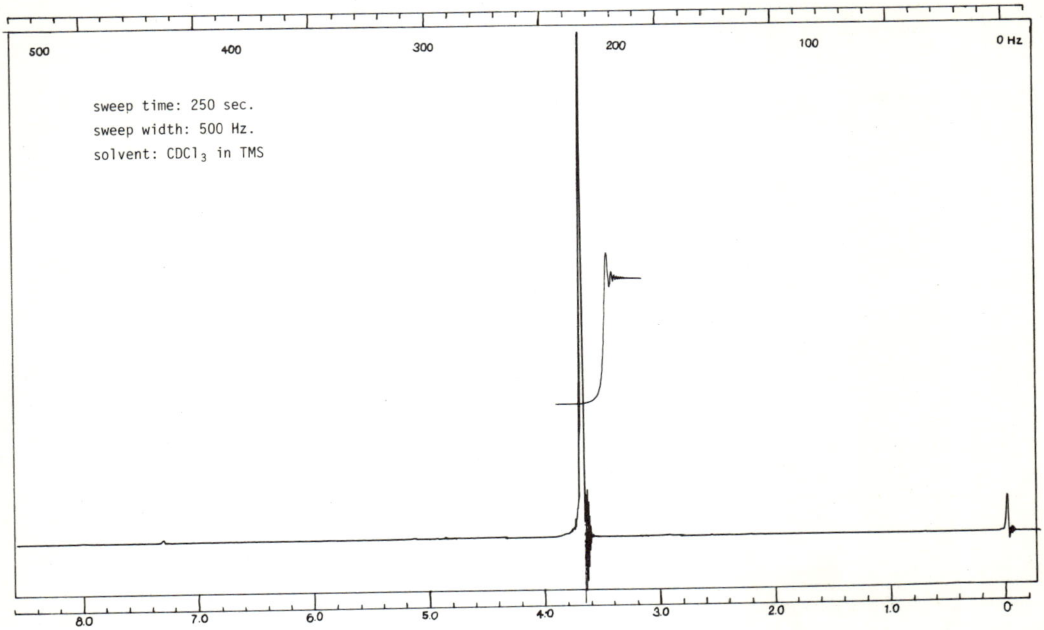
500
400
300
200
100
0 Hz
sweep time: 250 sec.
sweep width: 500 Hz.
solvent: CDCl3 in TMS
8.0
7.0
6.0
5.0
4.0
3.0
2.0
1.0
0

(d)

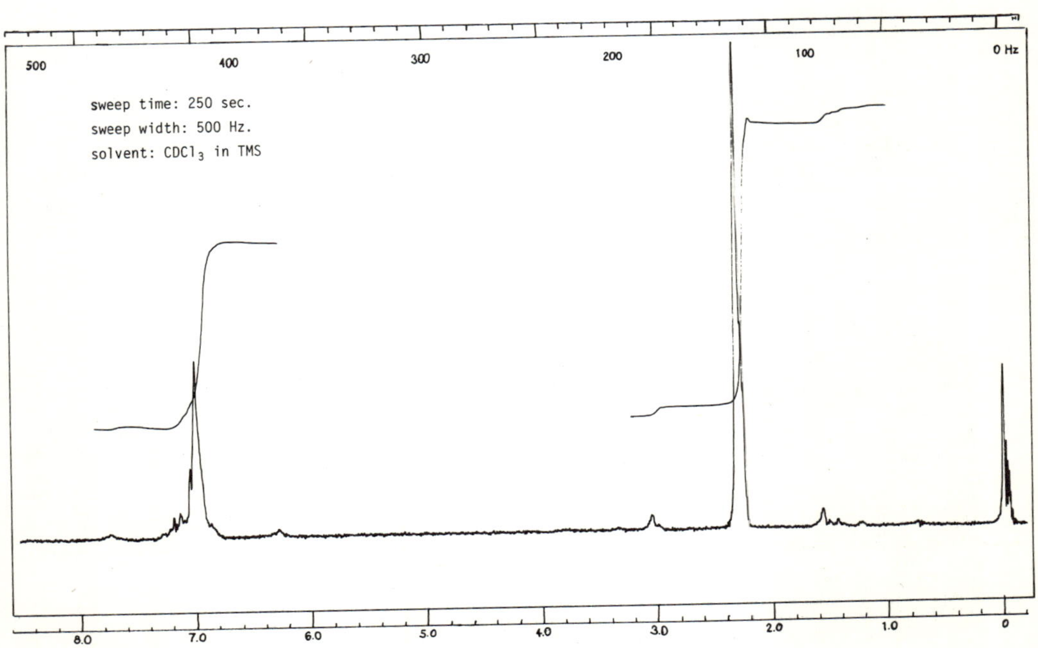
500
400
300
200
100
0 Hz
sweep time: 250 sec.
sweep width: 500 Hz.
solvent: CDCl3 in TMS
8.0
7.0
6.0
5.0
4.0
3.0
2.0
1.0
0

Chapter 14

XIV. Mass Spectrometry

The principles underlying mass spectrometry are different from those we have discussed in connection with the other spectroscopic methods. In mass spectrometry, a sample is bombarded with an electron beam to produce a series of positive ion fragments that are quantitatively recorded as the *mass spectrum*.

To obtain a mass spectrum, the sample under investigation is introduced into a vacuum chamber where it is vaporized. The gas is then leaked into an ionization chamber where it is bombarded with a beam of electrons. On collision, an electron transfers energy to a sample molecule. The energy transferred can be sufficient to produce a variety of products, including positive ions. These are accelerated out of the ion source, separated according to their respective masses (actually mass to charge ratio or m/e), and finally directed toward an ion collector. Ions striking the collector produce a flow of electrons proportional to ion abundance. These electrical signals are amplified and recorded to produce the spectrum. The horizontal axis or abscissa indicates the mass of the positive fragments while the ordinate or vertical axis indicates their relative abundance. The most intense peak in the spectrum is called the *base peak* and is arbitrarily set as equal to 100 percent.

Sample Ionization

The initial result of the electron interaction with the molecule is the formation of the *molecular ion* (often designated as M^+) by ejection of another electron. Part, sometimes essentially all, of the molecular ion decomposes further to the *fragment ions* of the spectrum. For example, the principal peaks in the spectrum of methanol are probably formed through the process:

$$CH_3OH + e \rightarrow CH_3OH^{+\cdot}\ (m/3 = 32) + 2e$$

$$CH_3OH^{+\cdot} \rightarrow CH_2OH^+\ (m/e = 31) + H^\cdot$$

$$\quad\longrightarrow CH_3^+\ (m/e = 15) + {}^\cdot OH$$

$$CH_2OH^+ \rightarrow CHO^+\ (m/e = 29) + H_2$$

Thus, methanol will have peaks in its spectrum corresponding to masses of 32 (molecular ion), 31, 29, and 15. Note that *only* the *positive* ion fragments appear in the spectrum; the hydrogen radical ($H^\cdot$), the hydrogen molecule (H_2), and the hydroxyl radical ($OH^\cdot$) will not appear.

In interpretation of the mass spectrum, identification of the molecular ion determines the *molecular weight* and often the elemental composition (C, H, O, N, etc.) of the molecule, and the interpreter attempts to deduce how these pieces fit together in the original molecular structure.

Determination of Molecular Formula

After one obtains the molecular weight of the sample from the mass of the molecular ion, it is desirable to determine its molecular formula or elemental composition. The most powerful technique for this utilizes the high-resolution mass spectrometer, a sophisticated and costly instrument. Alternatively, the presence of isotopes of known natural abundance offers a useful and simple method for determining the molecular formula from data supplied by less costly and more readily available unit-resolution mass spectrometers.

High resolution Mass Spectrometry. Determination of the exact mass of the molecular or fragment ions can define the elemental composition directly. The monoisotopic atomic weights of the elements are not exactly whole numbers on the basis of $^{12}C = 12.00000$, so that sufficiently careful mass measurements can distinguish between ions that weigh the same when weight is taken to the nearest whole number. For example, for an ion with unit mass weight of 28, there are four possible combinations of atoms:

$$CO = 27.9949 \qquad N_2 = 28.0062$$
$$CH_2N_2 = 28.0187 \qquad C_2H_4 = 28.0312$$

Thus, measurement of the mass to four decimal places makes it possible to distinguish between these four possibilities.

Natural Isotopic Abundances; Isotopic Clusters. Unit-resolution spectrometers that determine the mass of an ion to the nearest whole number are much more readily available than high-resolution mass spectrometers. With them one can rely on the relative intensities of *isotope peaks* to arrive at several possible molecular formulas. The final selection is then made on the basis of other evidence.

The mass spectrum of chemically pure carbon dioxide is a composite of the spectra of $^{12}C^{16}O_2$, $^{13}C^{16}O_2$, $^{12}C^{16}O^{18}O$, and so on. The molecular ions for these molecules are at 44, 45, and 46 respectively. Although the presence of this mixture makes the spectrum more complicated, the abundances of the isotopic components gives a direct indication of the elemental composition. Since for every 100 ^{12}C's in a sample there are 1.08 ^{13}C's, the peak at 45 will be approximately 1.08 percent of the intensity of the 44 peak. Remember that the mass spectrum is a record of the relative abundances of individual ions, and for a molecule like CO_2 with only one carbon atom, each one of these ions will contain either a ^{12}C or a ^{13}C but not both. Some elements have more than one isotope of appreciable natural abundance. A second isotope is especially prominent in the spectrum if it is more than one mass unit higher than the more abundant isotopic species. Bromine and chlorine and, to a lesser extent, silicon and sulfur are common examples. The presence of these elements in an ion is often easily recognized from the "isotopic clusters" produced in the spectrum. A sample containing bromine will give a mass spectrum that will have clusters of peaks two mass units apart, one due to an ion containing ^{79}Br and one due to an identical ion containing ^{81}Br, and these peaks will be in a 1:1 ratio. For our present purposes, it is sufficient to say that the elemental composition of an ion can be determined from isotope data in many cases. Further details of the process are beyond the scope of this course.

Degree of Unsaturation

Because of the valences of the elements involved, the total number of rings and double bonds (or unsaturated sites) in a molecule of the formula $C_xH_yN_zO_n$ will be equal to $x - 1/2y + 1/2z + 1$. Determination of the molecular formula thus gives the number of unsaturated sites in the molecule. This formula is useful in determining how the fragments go together.

Fragmentation

There are some general rules for predicting peaks in the mass spectrum of a given compound or for rationalizing peaks in the mass spectrum of an unknown. They are all based on the principle that the main fragment ion peaks of a compound should correspond to the most stable ion products of the most favorable reaction pathway. Six basic rules may be given.

1. In alkyl chains, cleavage (fragmentation) is favored at branched carbon atoms since tertiary and secondary carbonium ions are more stable than primary carbonium ions.

2. Aromatic rings, carbon-carbon double bonds, and nonaromatic rings stabilize the molecular ion (M^+) once it is formed and increase the probability of its prominent appearance in the spectrum.

3. Double bonds favor allylic cleavage:

$$R{-}CH_2CH{=}CH_2 \rightarrow R^{\cdot} + {}^{+}CH_2{-}CH{=}CH_2$$

4. In alkyl substituted aromatic compounds, cleavage to produce a benzylic type cation is favored:

$$C_6H_5CH_2{-}R \rightarrow C_6H_5CH_2^{+} + R^{\cdot}$$

5. Carbon-carbon bonds adjacent to heteroatoms (N, O, S) are frequently cleaved:

$$CH_3{-}CH_2{-}NH_2 \rightarrow CH_3^{\cdot} + CH_2{-}NH_2$$

6. Small stable neutral species are often eliminated during the formation of fragment ions. Examples are H_2O, CO, ethylene, and acetylene. When one of these neutral species is eliminated from a molecular ion, there will be a peak in the spectrum corresponding to the mass of the molecular ion minus the fragment.

Elimination of neutral molecules may be the result of a rearrangement of which the best known example is the *McLafferty rearrangement*. This involves the rearrangement of a hydrogen atom to a polar functional group of an ion:

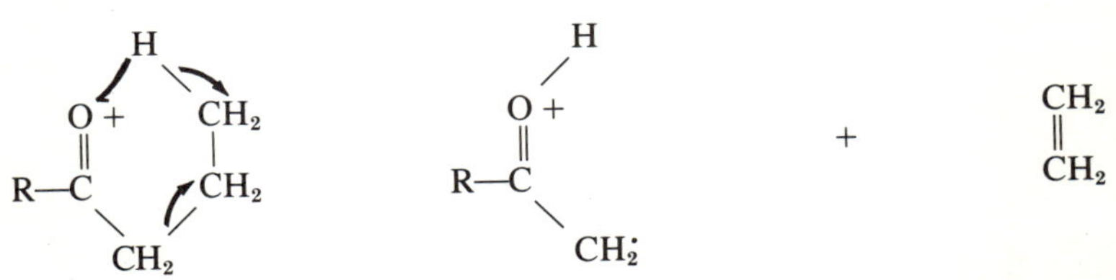

$[M\text{-}28]^+$

It occurs often in aldehydes (R = H), ketones (R = alkyl or aryl), esters (R = O—R′), and acids (R = OH).

These rules do not cover all of the possible fragmentation patterns, but they do cover many that common drug molecules undergo in the mass spectrometer and, with a little thought, they can be used to interpret the spectra of many simple drugs for the purposes of identification.

Experiment 17. Use of Spectroscopy for the Identification of Unknowns.

The identification of an unknown substance, whether in dosage forms or body fluids, is often facilitated by a study of its ultraviolet, infrared, nuclear magnetic resonance, and mass spectra. Depending on the availability of the instruments and class size, some instructors may wish to give students "hands-on" experience with these methods. The following experiment is an alternative if such experience is not feasible.

After appropriate demonstration of the instruments involved, students are given a set of spectra for one of the following compounds (see Appendix):

acetaminophen
acetanilid
antipyrine
benzocaine
benzyl benzoate
chlordiazepoxide (HCl)
p-dimethylaminobenzaldehyde
diphenhydramine
menthyl salicylate
phenyl salicylate
sulfanilamide
theophylline

Look up the structures of these compounds. Speculate on the nature of the spectra they should produce. When you have received an unknown number, analyze its spectrum carefully and report the identity of your "unknown", indicating the specific spectral characteristics which led you to your conclusion.

PROBLEMS

1. The four most intense peaks in the mass spectrum of amphetamine

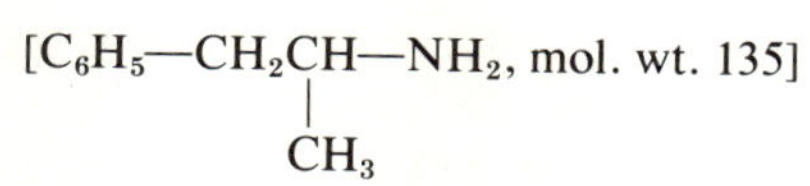

occur at masses of 120, 91, 65, and 44. Give the structures of the fragment ions.

2. Methadone is represented by the following structure:

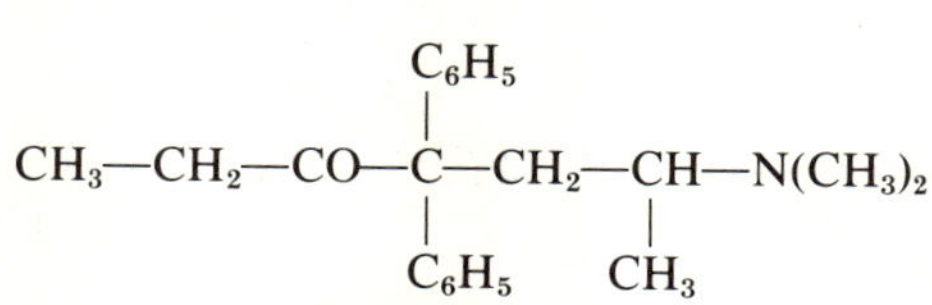

Show four of the fragment ions expected in the mass spectrum.

3. Four compounds all having the same molecular formula $C_9H_{10}O$ are shown:

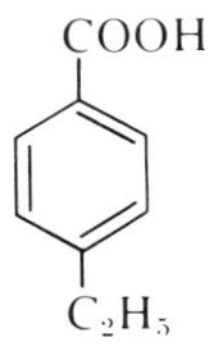
I

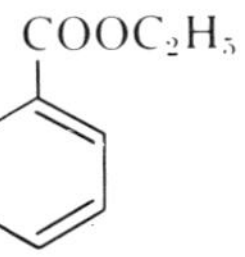
II

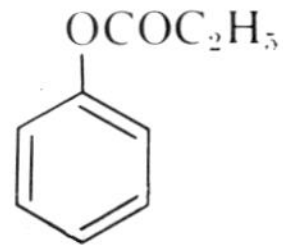
III

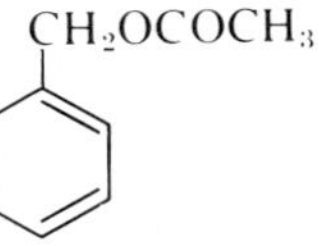
IV

Distinctions between them can be made on the basis of their mass spectra. Indicate which of the compounds fulfills each of the conditions a through e. One of the compounds has:

(a) prominent fragment ions at 133 and 105.
(b) an initial fragment of mass 105 which fragments further to give an ion of mass 77 and carbon monoxide.
(c) a fragment ion of mass 43 containing oxygen.
(d) a distinctive fragment ion of mass 57.
(e) a fragment ion of mass 91 which loses ethylene to give an ion of mass 65.

ANSWERS

3. (a) I
   (b) II
   (c) IV
   (d) III
   (e) IV

Chapter 15

Atomic Absorption Spectroscopy

One other spectroscopic method deserves mention for its application in the detection of small amounts of metals—as in the determination of lead in paint residues, mercury in fish, toxic metals in biological samples, and the like. This method is known as atomic absorption spectroscopy. It uses a flame to excite metal atoms from their ground states.

The instrument includes a hollow cathode lamp as a light source. The light it supplies is characteristic of the metal of the cathode used in the manufacture of the lamp. The cathode metal is chosen specifically for the metal to be analyzed. A burner produces a flame into which a fine spray of solution is nebulized. Finally, a monochromator-detector is used to separate the flame and the solution spectra and record the spectrum of the metal of interest.

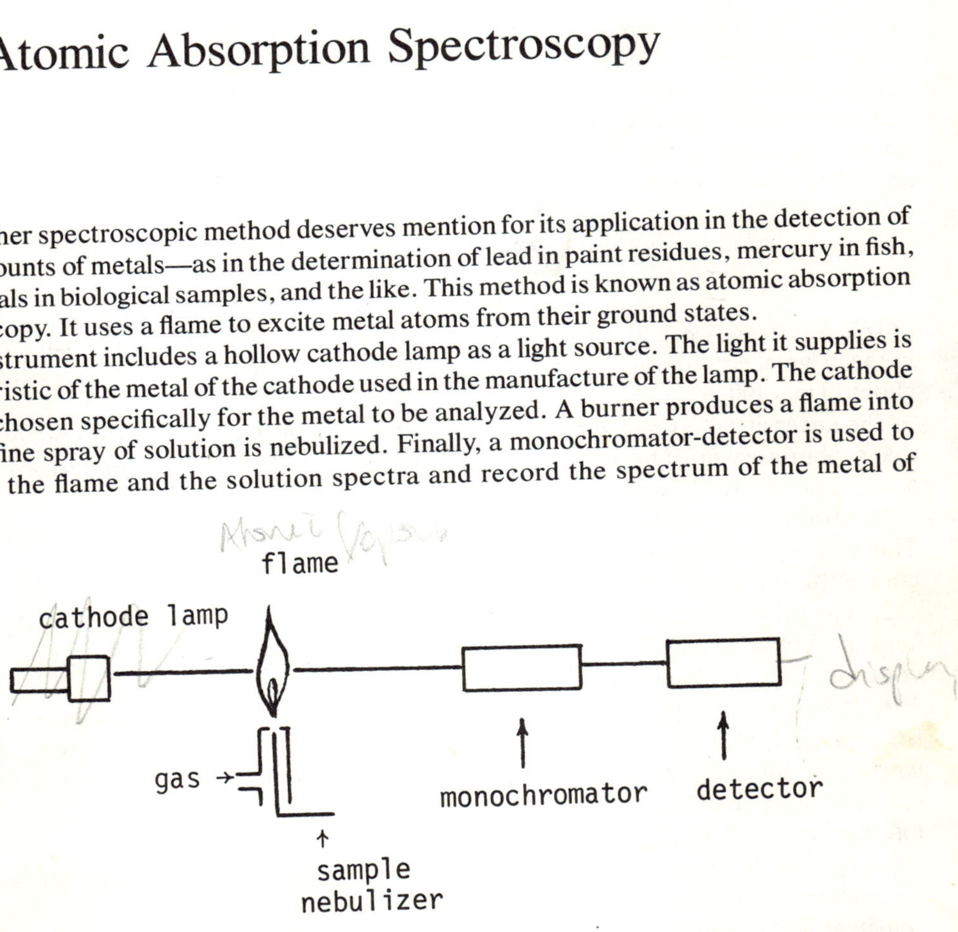

In practice the sample solution is sprayed into the flame (2000 to 3500° K.) which serves to volatilize the solvent and dissociate the salt into its free atoms in the ground state. Light from the cathode lamp enters the flame and part of it is absorbed by the sample atoms resulting in the excitation of their valence electrons. When these electrons drop back to their ground states, a photon of light is given off. The absorption and emission by the metal atoms in the flame changes the unidirectional light of the cathode lamp to multidirectional light, i.e., it is scattered, whereby a portion of the absorbed light escapes the detector. The intensity of the light beam decreases accordingly; the higher the concentration of substance in the flame, the less light gets through to the detector. In the *absence* of appropriate ions in the flame, light from the cathode lamp simply passes through the flame into the monochromator-detector where it is separated from the flame spectrum and recorded.

Modern instruments record the data as peaks representing the log of light intensity. Signal peaks, similar to those seen in gas chromatography, are obtained. In addition, the scale is reversed so that high readings are obtained for high concentrations. Since in typical use an operator would plot the peak height vs. concentration for a number of known standards prior to measuring the unknown concentration, this results in a low reading for the blank and increasing readings for successively increasing concentrations. This modification results in greater technician acceptance.

A further abbreviation of the procedure may be accomplished by comparison of peak heights of sample vs. standard as was done for gas chromatography (p. 75). For example, when a properly treated serum sample (5 ml.) was prepared for Ca^{++} assay, it was diluted 1:20 and its absorption determined, giving a peak height of 22.5 cm. A Ca^{++} standard containing 0.50 mg./100 ml. gave a peak height of 24.8 cm. The subsequent calculation should be easy to follow:

$$\frac{[Ca^{++}] \text{ in unknown}}{\text{peak height of unknown}} = \frac{[Ca^{++}] \text{ in standard}}{\text{peak height of standard}}$$

or $x/22.5 = 0.50/24.8$, and $x = 0.45$ mg./100 ml. Since a dilution of 1:20 was involved, $[Ca^{++}]$ in the original serum was 20 times this or 9 mg./100 ml. The normal serum calcium level is about 10 mg./100 ml.

The necessity of using a different cathode lamp for each element to be analyzed means that a laboratory must have a number of these lamps on hand. In addition, there are a few sources of interference in the method:

1. Absorption by solid particles or unvaporized solvent in the flame may be a problem. This can happen when too much solution is aspirated into the flame or when the salt concentration is too high.

2. The presence of easily ionized elements will add free electrons to the system and supress ionization of the atom of interest. This may be overcome by adding the same concentration of the interfering ion to both standards and sample.

3. Refractory compounds may be formed in the flame through reaction of an anion with the cation of interest. Normally this can be prevented by adding enough strontium or lanthanum chloride to make the solution about 1 percent in these ions. Sr^{++} and La^{3+} will react with the interfering anion making it unavailable for reaction with the element of interest in the determination.

As against these seeming disadvantages, atomic absorption is generally subject to less interference, for example, than flame photometry, and is quite sensitive, almost too sensitive, in the routine analysis of metal containing drugs. Common levels of detection include Na, 0.03; Mg, 0.001; Ca, 0.08; Zn, 0.0005; and Pb, 0.013 p.p.m. The method finds utility in fields ranging from clinical chemistry to geology.

In occupational health studies, biological samples such as blood, urine, or tissue are often analyzed by atomic absorption spectroscopy. Normally such samples are ashed to destroy organic matter, or wet-ashed by digesting repeatedly with concentrated nitric acid and evaporating to dryness. The residue is then dissolved in hydrochloric acid and diluted with distilled, deionized water prior to analysis. In patients being treated for lead poisoning by calcium EDTA, the need for ashing is eliminated inasmuch as the urine need only be diluted to reduce high salt content prior to analysis. Pharmaceuticals that contain metal ions can be analyzed by atomic absorption. For example, it has been used for the analysis of Ringer's solution (Na, K, Ca); by simply changing cathode lamps, these three ions can be determined in a single procedure* whereas the U.S.P. assay (XIX, 443) requires three separate titrimetric procedures.

PROBLEMS

1. A serum sample is to be assayed for lithium levels to determine the blood levels required for therapeutic activity. Standards containing 2, 4, 6, 8, 10, and 12 p.p.m. lithium were analyzed, and the results indicated a straight line relationship between peak heights and concentration. When a serum sample was diluted 1:5 and then injected, it gave a peak height of 2.5 cm. as compared to 9.7 cm. for the 8 p.p.m. standard. Calculate the serum lithium concentration.
2. The zinc levels in Globin Zinc Insulin Injection (U.S.P. XIX, 254) may be determined using atomic absorption. A vial containing 100 U. was diluted 1:100 with hydrochloric acid and trichloroacetic acid, centrifuged, and a portion of this sample diluted 1:1000. Atomic absorption gave a peak of 18.9 cm. as compared to 15.4 cm. for the 3 p.p.m. standard. Calculate the concentration of zinc in milligrams per 100 U.

ANSWERS

1. 10.3 p.p.m.
2. 0.37 mg./100 U.

*Smith, R. V., and Nessen, M. A.: *Atomic absorption analysis of sodium, potassium and calcium in Ringer's solution*. J. Pharm. Sci. 60:907, 1971.

Chapter 16

Miscellaneous Methods

A number of other analytical methods have been developed primarily for their clinical application, and it is appropriate to mention a few of these for the health professional with interests in that direction. A group of related procedures including (1) separation in gels, (2) immunoelectrophoresis, (3) radioimmunoassay, (4) agglutination, (5) immunofluorescence, and (6) enzyme immunoassay have been applied to the detection of trace amounts of chemicals in biological fluids. Of these, radioimmunoassay, enzyme immunoassay, and electrophoresis have been developed into extremely useful methods for the qualitative and quantitative assay of low levels of drugs and other physiologically active compounds.

RADIOIMMUNOASSAY (RIA)

A radioimmunoassay begins with an injection into animals of a drug or chemical which has been covalently bound to a macromolecule. This drug-macromolecule complex is recognized by the animal body as foreign, and antibody formation results. After repeated injections of the drug-macromolecule complex, the animals are bled and the antibodies are collected. These will now bind in vitro with the parent drug molecule. This in vitro drug-antibody interaction forms the basis for radioimmunoassay. In the assay, a known quantity of radioactive drug is added to the antibody solution and the "unknown" serum sample is added to the mixture. If the particular drug of interest is present in the serum, the following competitive reaction occurs (asterisk denotes radioactivity):

$$\text{Drug} + \text{Drug}^{*} + \text{Antibody} \leftrightarrows \text{Drug-Antibody} + \text{Drug}^{*}\text{-Antibody}$$

The amount of radioactive drug that is not bound to the antibody is determined. The quantity of this free radioactive drug is proportional to the level of the drug in the serum. The method will readily detect picogram (10^{-12} gm.) quantities of low molecular weight substances. Normally, standard curves are generated by using solutions of different concentrations in the region of interest. A plot, on semi-log paper, of drug concentration vs. percent drug bound looks like that shown in the figure on p. 142. The serum concentration may then be determined by reading directly from the standard curve.

Prepared kits containing the necessary reagents are commercially available. For drugs, the assays use ^{125}I-labelled antigens which have a half-life of 60 days; therefore the kits have

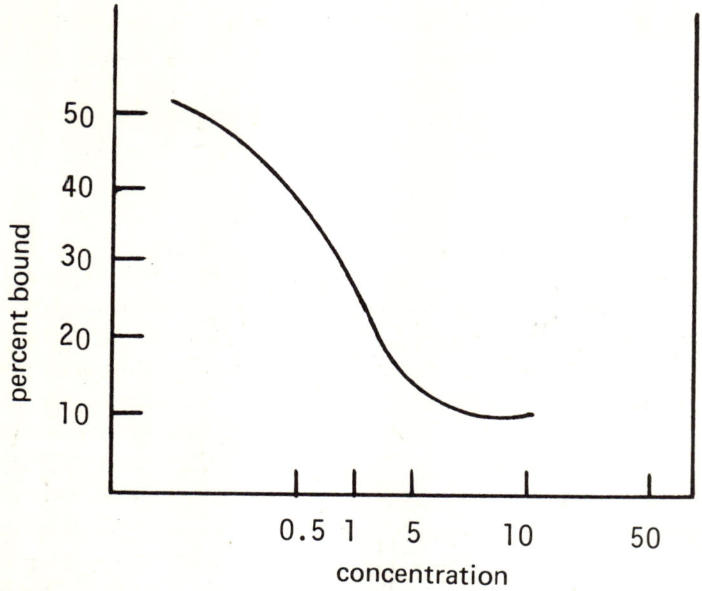

a reasonable shelf life of 2 to 4 months. The assays require 30 min. to 1 hr. to complete and sample sizes of 0.1 μl. or less. Urinary concentrations can be detected reliably at levels between 100 μg./L. (morphine, barbiturates, methadone, methaqualone) and 1000 μg./L. (amphetamine). Antibody-coated beads and test tubes have become available recently; these greatly simplify the assay. For example, a serum sample is added directly to the test tube, followed by the tracer reagent. The combination is allowed to incubate for a prescribed period and then the solution is removed and the test tube subjected to a radioactive count. This process eliminates the sensitive precipitation step common to most RIA procedures. Because the antibody is bound to the test tube, less care is required in the decantation or aspiration step.

The types of drugs for which kits for this modification of the method are available include digoxin, digitoxin, methotrexate, lysergic acid diethylamide (LSD), and ouabain. In addition, kits are available for a number of other physiologically active substances including renin, aldosterone, insulin, growth hormone, thyroxine, triiodothyronine, folic acid, and vitamin B_{12}.

ENZYME IMMUNOASSAY

This process involves the covalent labelling of an enzyme with an antibody, hapten, or antigen. In the case of drugs, an antibody-reactive drug derivative is bound to an enzyme. When antibodies to the drug are added, they interact with the drug-enzyme complex, changing the enzyme conformation and modifying its activity. It is this change in enzyme activity that is used as an indirect measure of the presence of the drug. For example, when the serum containing this drug is exposed to the drug-enzyme-antibody complex, the free drug and the enzyme-bound drug compete for the antibody, resulting in less antibody being bound to the drug-enzyme. The advantages of this method over radioimmunoassay include: (1) relatively inexpensive equipment is required, (2) the method has a potential for automation, (3) there are no radiation hazards, and (4) the shelf life of the reagents is not limited by radioactive decay (^{125}I has a half-life of 60 days).

Commercial kits are available for the analysis of phenytoin, phenobarbi carbamazepine, ethosuximide, digoxin, amphetamine, propoxyphene, benzo metabolite, cocaine metabolite, and methadone. These assays have their principal application in the clinical laboratory. Further details can be obtained from some recently published works, by Cleeland and coworkers,* Scharpe and coworkers,† and Wisdom.‡

ELECTROPHORESIS

Electrophoresis is a separation technique which, like chromatography, can involve a column or paper support to which the sample is applied. Instead of gravity, pump pressure, or gas stream, movement of the sample and eventual separation are based on the effect of an electric field on the charged species in solution. Often the sample is applied midway between the two poles. As electrophoresis proceeds, the negatively charged components migrate toward the anode, the positively charged components toward the cathode. Many support materials can be used to carry out electrophoretic separations including chromatography paper, starch gel, Sephadex, cellulose acetate, and polyacrylamide gels. The use of these last supports has become very popular because they show decreased convection and diffusion effects. In carrying out electrophoretic separations, buffers are normally used to control pH. A typical system using paper or a cellulose acetate strip can be described schematically as shown in the figure below.

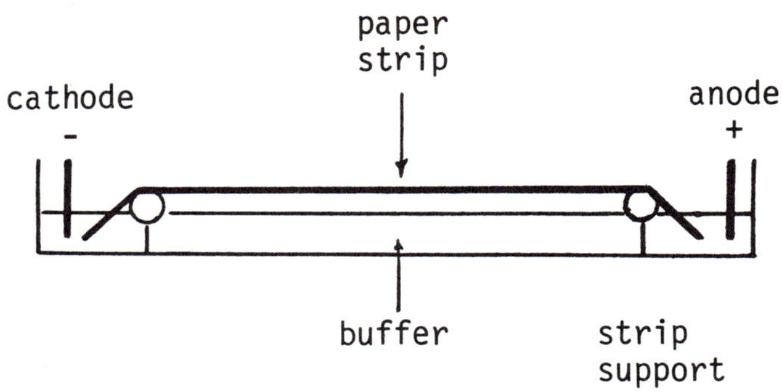

During a strip separation, heat buildup can be a problem. If the strip becomes hot, the buffer may evaporate and the sample can be destroyed. To prevent this, the current is kept low and the buffer is refrigerated before use. A second complication involves movement of the sample, independent of its ionic character, by being carried along with the solvent. To compensate for this, a nonpolar marker can be added to the sample. If the nonpolar marker moves, its movement is subtracted from the sample movement.

To obtain qualitative information concerning the components present in a mixture, a standard solution is normally run along with the unknown. In this way, one can detect the presence or absence of any abnormal polar substances. In addition to knowing what is present, it is often desirable to know how much is present. One way of doing this is to cut out the spots, elute them, and determine the concentration of the substances by

---

*Cleeland, R., et al.: *Detection of drugs of abuse by radioimmunoassay: A summary of published data and some new information.* Clin. Chem. 22:712, 1976.

†Scharpe, S. L., et al.: *Quantitative enzyme immunoassay: Current status.* Clin. Chem. 22:733, 1976.

‡Wisdom, G. B.: *Enzyme immunoassay.* Clin. Chem. 22:1243, 1976.

spectroscopic methods. An easier and more widely used approach involves use of a densitometer, the absorbence of the different regions on the strip are measured and peaks, which are plots of absorbence vs. position on the strip, are obtained from the recorder. The areas under the peaks are proportional to the concentration of the substances responsible for them.

Electrophoresis has limited potential in traditional drug analysis, but it is widely used in clinical chemistry. Separations of substances such as serum proteins, lipoproteins, glycoprotein, hemoglobin, and haptoglobin are commonly accomplished by this means.

Chapter 17

Putting It All Together

A variety of problems of pharmaceutical importance depend for their solution not on the utilization of a single analytical technique but on a combination of several of the methods we have considered in this course. To conclude this introduction to drug analysis, it seems appropriate to illustrate such combinations by brief reference to at least two types of problems in which they have been used successfully.

Because alkaloids are often pharmacologically active constituents of plants, research in schools of pharmacy and in the pharmaceutical industry is often directed to a study of these compounds. Such an investigation led, a few years ago, to the discovery of alkaloids in the leaves of the maple *Acer saccharinum,* and for the sake of example, we can reconstruct the series of events which might have been involved in their isolation and identification.

Alcohol is an excellent solvent for a wide variety of naturally occurring organic substances including many which we use as drugs. An alcoholic extract, after removal of the solvent, presents a complex mixture of compounds which is usually separated by SOLVENT EXTRACTION. In the present case, partition between ether and dilute aqueous ammonia was used to extract the alkaloids, as their free bases, into the organic phase. Further purification was achieved by further extraction of the ether phase with dilute acid and reprecipitation of the alkaloid(s) with base. The principle is similar to that described on page 69. It was not necessary to determine the PARTITION COEFFICIENT in this case; extractions were repeated several times to insure quantitative removal of the desired product(s). The residue was weighed to estimate the percentage of alkaloid in the plant.

A small portion of the crude mixture was subjected to THIN LAYER CHROMATOGRAPHY exactly as described in Experiment 11, page 79, using Dragendorff's reagent to visualize the spots. This suggested the presence of one major component along with traces of three impurities. COLUMN CHROMATOGRAPHY using alumina as an adsorbent and the GRADIENT ELUTION TECHNIQUE (page 73) resulted in the isolation of the single major component as a crystalline substance melting at 138°C. It showed no OPTICAL ROTATION. Combustion analysis indicated a molecular formula of $C_{11}H_{14}N_2$. The ULTRAVIOLET ABSORPTION SPECTRUM of an ethanol solution showed maxima at 217 and 280 nm. with $\epsilon = 37750$ and 6275 respectively. The INFRARED SPECTRUM exhibited bands at 2.9, 3.4, 3.6, 9.8, and 12.2μ. (For practice, see if you can assign these bands to their functional groups). An NMR SPECTRUM gave the following data:

δ(p.p.m.)	*Splitting*	*Integration*	*Interpretation*
7.2	multiplet	4	aromatic protons
7.4	multiplet	1	NH of indole
6.8	singlet	1	α-H of indole
3.0	singlet	2	$—CH_2—$
2.25	singlet	6	CH_3 on N

All of these data serve to identify the compound as gramine (see below), an alkaloid which had been reported previously only from certain grasses. This was its first appearance in maples.* It has since been isolated also from certain species of legumes. Gramine is a smooth muscle stimulant but has no known medical use.

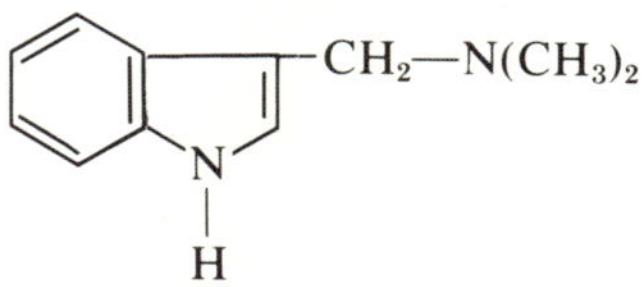

Another example of the use of these combined techniques is found in the application of analytical methods to the detection and identification of drugs in patients suspected of drug abuse or overdose. It often happens in such cases that the amount of material retrievable from drug residues or body fluids is relatively small, and for this reason almost all of the methods to which we have referred have been adapted to the rapid detection of small amounts of drug. In most cases concentration of the ingredients sought in, for example, urine or serum, is accomplished by absorption on RESIN EXCHANGERS followed by elution, with BUFFERED SOLUTIONS, to achieve a degree of separation at the same time. Thus, morphine is removed from urine by absorption on a small column of Amberlite resin and eluted therefrom by a borate buffer at pH = 9.3. Suitable manipulation of the aqueous phase allows isolation of the morphine by SOLVENT EXTRACTION into an organic phase which, on concentration, yields the drug. Depending on the availability of equipment and analytical expertise, as well as on the amount of drug recovered, several methods have been used for its estimation. Color tests, relatively specific for opiate narcotics, can give presumptive evidence of their presence. Confirmation by THIN LAYER CHROMATOGRAPHY, GAS CHROMATOGRAPHY, or INFRARED SPECTROSCOPY have been used, along with quantitation by gas chromatography and ULTRAVIOLET SPECTROSCOPY. In selected laboratories where the very sophisticated gas chromatograph-mass spectrometer combination is available, the MASS SPECTRUM of a sample suspected to be morphine can be compared, with reference to its fragment ions, to a standard sample of the drug.

It is not to be expected, of course, that the average practicing pharmacist be able to do such determinations. But it has been suggested that knowledge of the methods, their applications, their limitations, and the availability of competent analysts in his community is a legitimate, and sometimes important, part of his professional contribution to the people he serves.

*Pachter, I. J., Zacharias, D. E., and Ribeiro, O.: *Indole alkaloids of Acer saccharinum, Dictyoloma incanescens, Piptadenia colubrina and Mimosa hostilis*. J. Am. Pharm. Assoc. 48:670, 1959.

Appendix

ATOMIC WEIGHT TABLE (abbreviated)

Relative to C = 12.00

Aluminum	Al	26.98	Lead	Pb	207.19
Antimony	Sb	121.75	Lithium	Li	6.94
Arsenic	As	74.92	Magnesium	Mg	24.31
Barium	Ba	137.34	Mercury	Hg	200.59
Bismuth	Bi	208.98	Molybdenum	Mo	95.94
Boron	B	10.81	Nickel	Ni	58.78
Bromine	Br	79.91	Nitrogen	N	14.01
Cadmium	Cd	112.40	Oxygen	O	16.00
Calcium	Ca	40.08	Phosphorus	P	30.97
Carbon	C	12.01	Potassium	K	39.10
Cerium	Ce	140.12	Silicon	Si	28.09
Chlorine	Cl	35.45	Silver	Ag	107.87
Chromium	Cr	52.00	Sodium	Na	22.99
Cobalt	Co	58.93	Strontium	Sr	87.62
Copper	Cu	63.54	Sulfur	S	32.06
Fluorine	F	19.00	Tin	Sn	118.69
Hydrogen	H	1.01	Titanium	Ti	47.90
Iodine	I	126.90	Vanadium	V	50.94
Iron	Fe	55.85	Zinc	Zn	65.37

TABLE OF IONIZATION CONSTANTS

Acids

Acetic	1.75×10^{-5}
Benzoic	6.3×10^{-5}
Boric	6.4×10^{-10}

TABLE OF IONIZATION CONSTANTS

Acids

Carbonic	$4.3 \times 10^{-7}, 4.8 \times 10^{-11}$
EDTA	$1.0 \times 10^{-2}, 2.2 \times 10^{-3}, 6.9 \times 10^{-7}, 5.5 \times 10^{-11}$
Lactic	1.4×10^{-4}
Oxalic	$6.5 \times 10^{-2}, 6.1 \times 10^{-5}$
Phenol	1.1×10^{-10}
Phthalic (*ortho*)	$1.2 \times 10^{-3}, 3.9 \times 10^{-6}$
Salicylic	1.0×10^{-3}

Bases

Ammonia	1.75×10^{-5}
Diethylamine	8.5×10^{-4}
Ethanolamine	3.2×10^{-5}
Ethylenediamine	$8.5 \times 10^{-5}, 7.1 \times 10^{-8}$
Pyridine	1.7×10^{-9}
Tris (hydroxymethyl)-aminomethane	1.2×10^{-6}

SOLUBILITY PRODUCT CONSTANTS

Aluminum	$Al(OH)_3$	5.0×10^{-33}
Barium	$BaCO_3$	8.1×10^{-9}
	BaF_2	$1.7 \times 10_{-6}$
	$BaSO_4$	1.3×10^{-10}
Iron	$Fe(OH)_3$	1.1×10^{-36}
Lead	$PbCl_2$	1.6×10^{-5}
	$PbCrO_4$	1.8×10^{-14}
	PbS	4.2×10^{-28}
	$PbSO_4$	1.1×10^{-8}
Magnesium	$Mg(OH)_2$	3.4×10^{-11}
	$Mg(NH_4)PO_4$	3.0×10^{-13}
Silver	$AgCl$	1.56×10^{-10}
	Ag_2CrO_4	1.1×10^{-12}
	$AgCNS$	1.0×10^{-12}
	Ag_3PO_4	1.2×10^{-10}
	$AgIO_3$	3.1×10^{-8}

TABLE OF REDUCTION POTENTIALS

Reaction	E°, Volts
$MnO_4^- + 8\,H^+ + 5e \leftrightarrow Mn^{++} + 4\,H_2O$	+1.51
$Cl_2 + 2e \leftrightarrow 2\,Cl^-$	+1.36
$Cr_2O_7^= + 14\,H^+ + 6e \leftrightarrow 2\,Cr^{3+} + 7\,H_2O$	+1.33
$2\,IO_3^- + 12\,H^+ + 10e \leftrightarrow I_2 + 6\,H_2O$	+1.19
$Br_2 + 2e \leftrightarrow 2\,Br^-$	+1.09
$2\,Hg^{++} + 2e \leftrightarrow Hg_2^{++}$	+0.907
$Ag^+ + e \leftrightarrow Ag^\circ$	+0.799
$Fe^{3+} + e \leftrightarrow Fe{+}{+}$	+0.771
$O_2 + 2\,H^+ + 2e \leftrightarrow H_2O_2$	+0.682
$H_3AsO_4 + 2\,H^+ + 2e \leftrightarrow H_3AsO_3 + H_2O$	+0.559
$I_2 + 2e \leftrightarrow 2\,I^-$	+0.536
$Cu^{++} + 2e \leftrightarrow Cu^\circ$	+0.337
$S_4O_6^= + 2e \leftrightarrow 2\,S_2O_3^=$	+0.09
$2\,H^+ + 2e \leftrightarrow H_2$	0.000
$Pb^{++} + 2e \leftrightarrow Pb^\circ$	−0.126
$PbSO_4 + 2e \leftrightarrow Pb^\circ + SO_4^=$	−0.356
$2\,CO_2 + 2\,H^+ + 2e \leftrightarrow H_2C_2O_4$	−0.49
$Zn^{++} + 2e \leftrightarrow Zn^\circ$	−0.763

SPECTRA

The spectra reproduced on the following pages are those of the compounds suggested as "unknowns" in Experiment 17 (page 134). Use them to establish the structure of your unknown, and as practice, try to interpret the spectra of the other compounds on the list.

Compound No. 1

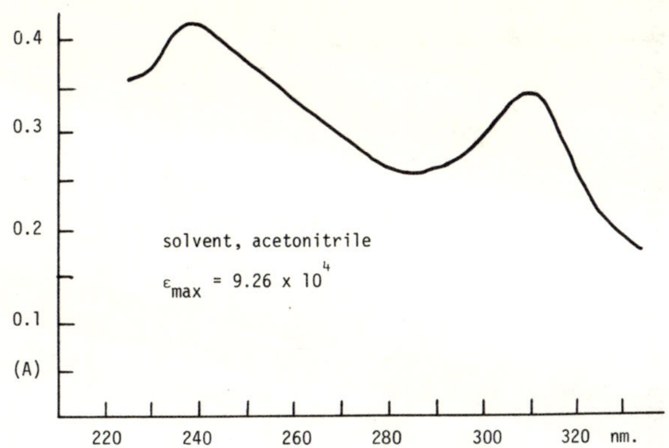

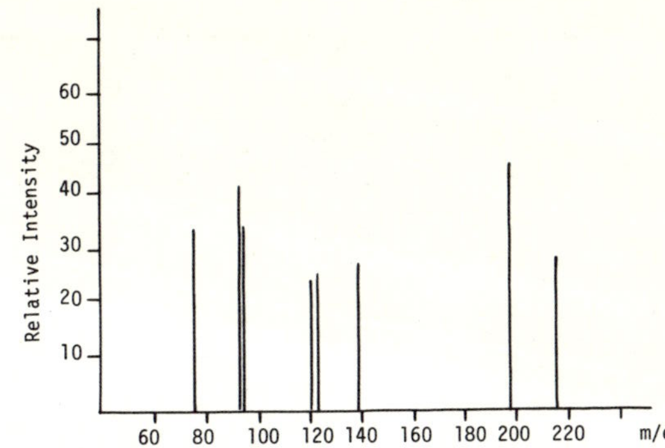

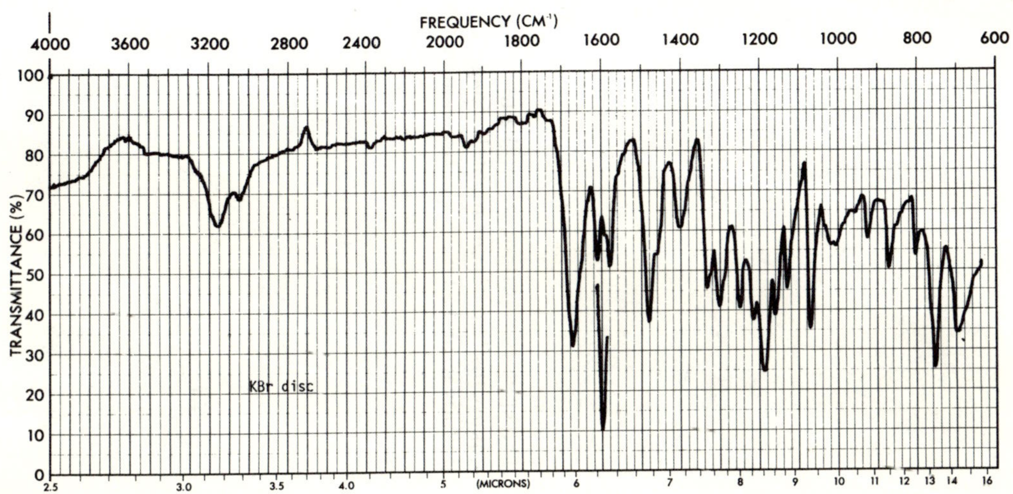

Compound No. 1

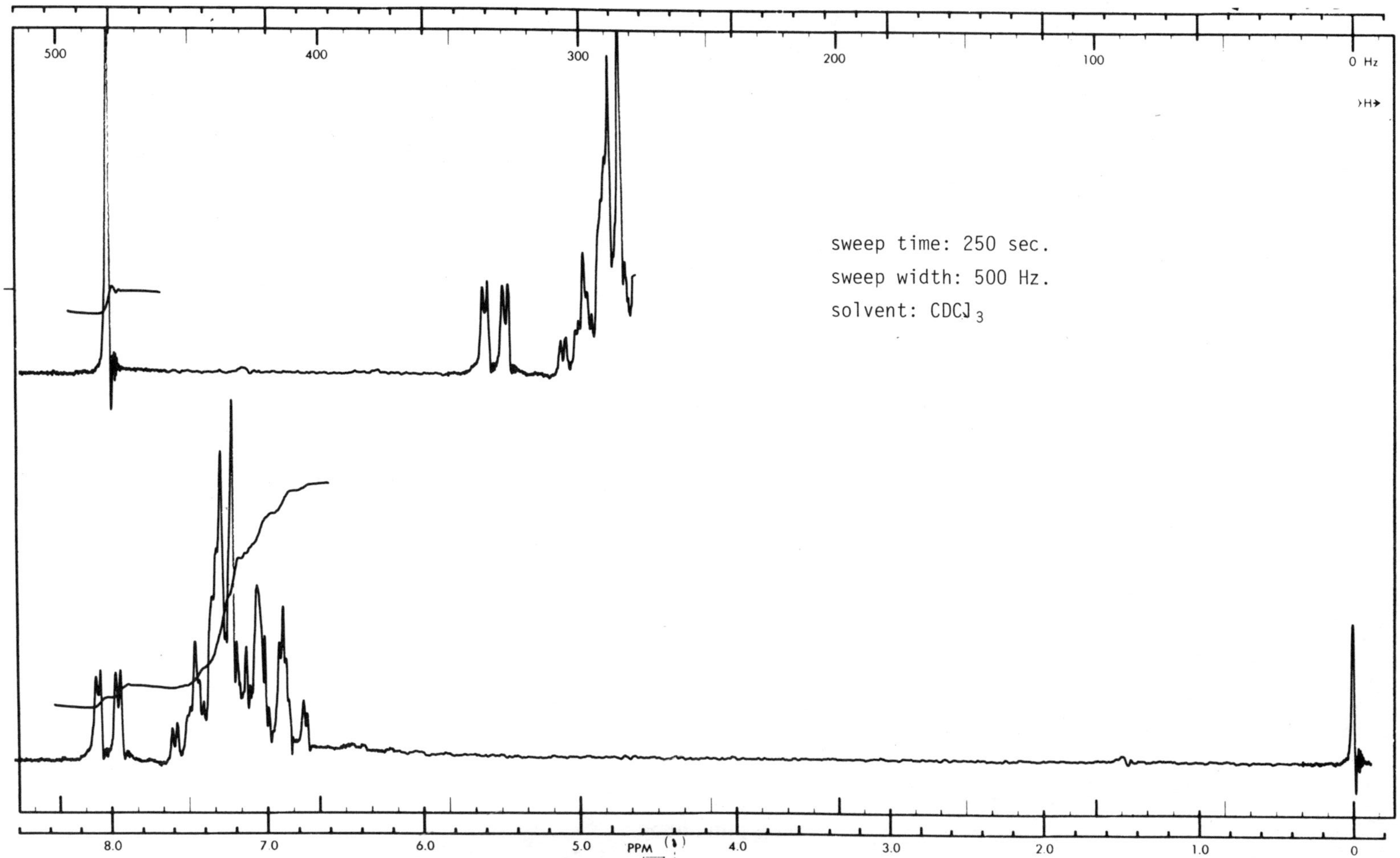

Compound No. 2

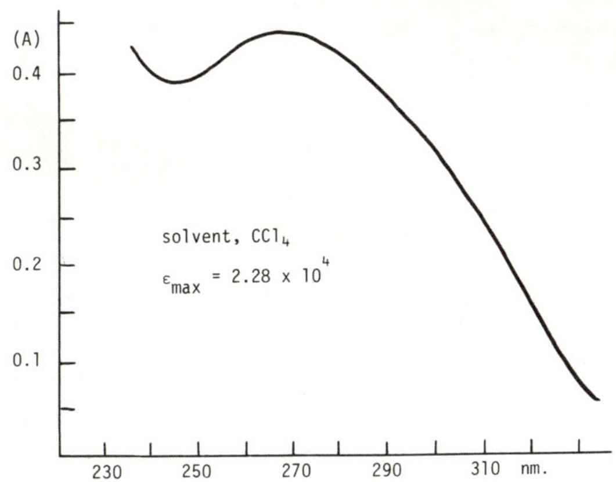

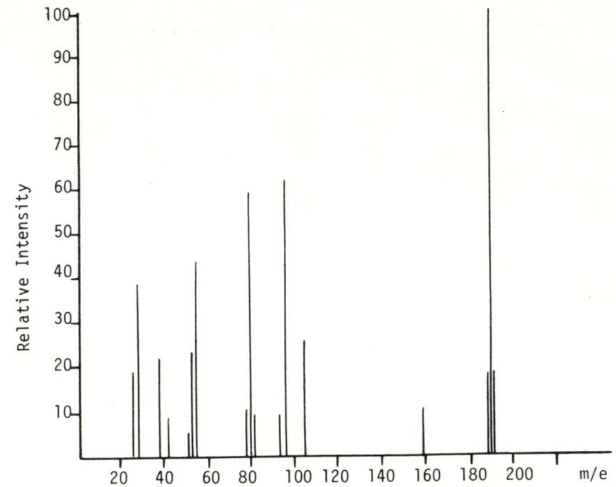

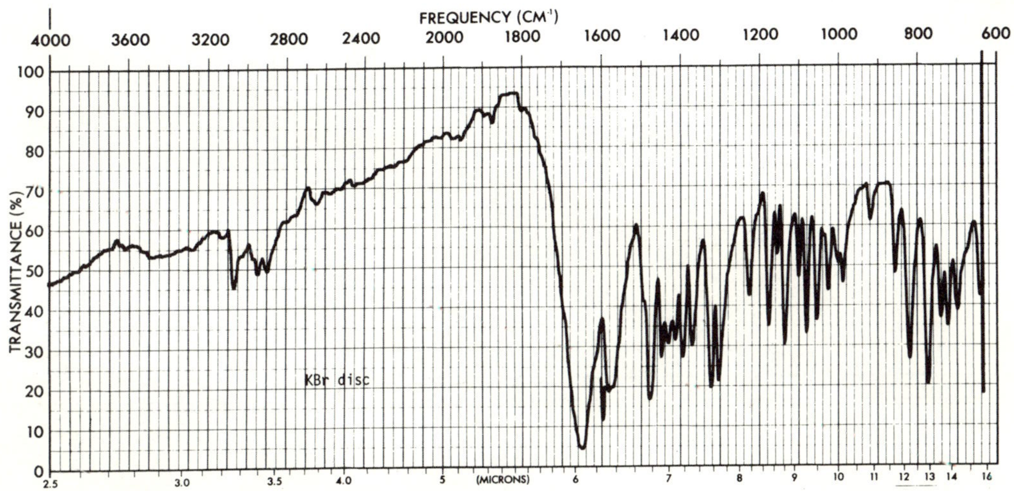

Compound No. 2

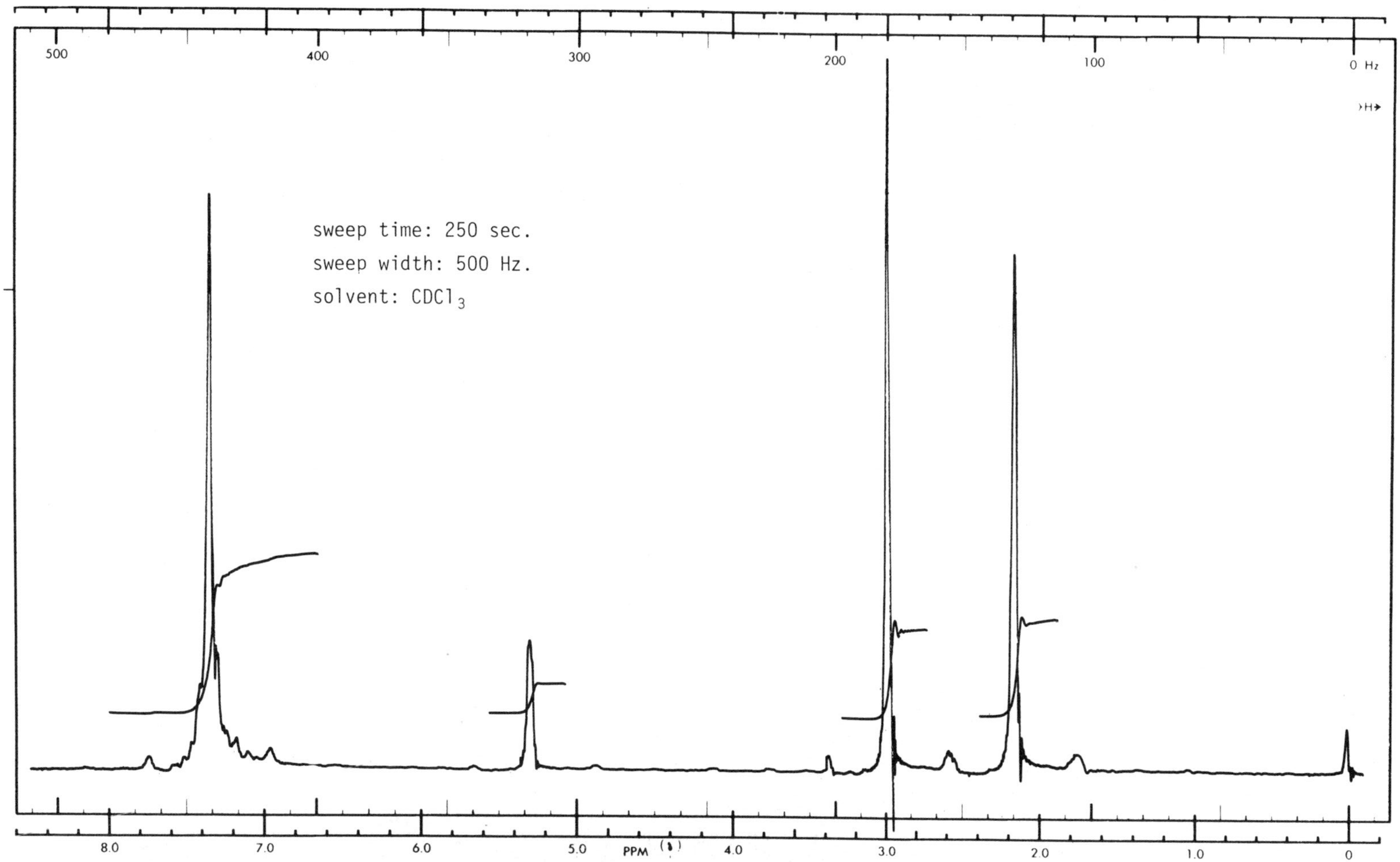

Compound No. 3

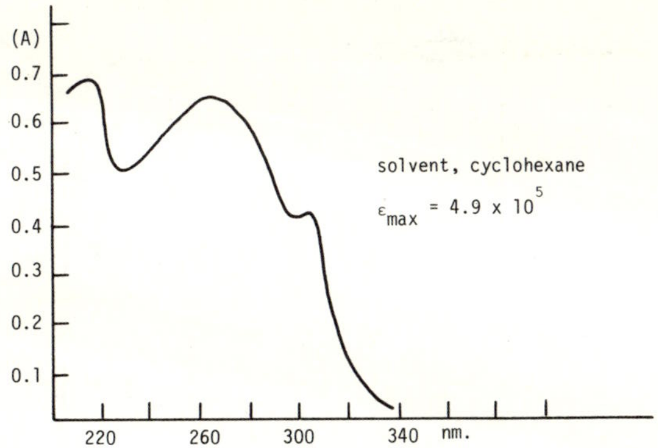

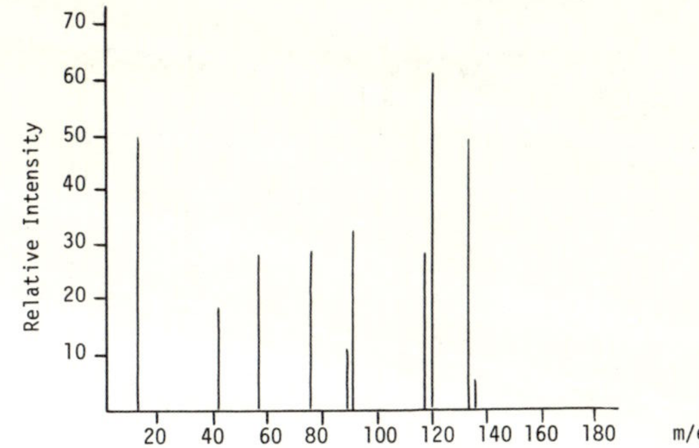

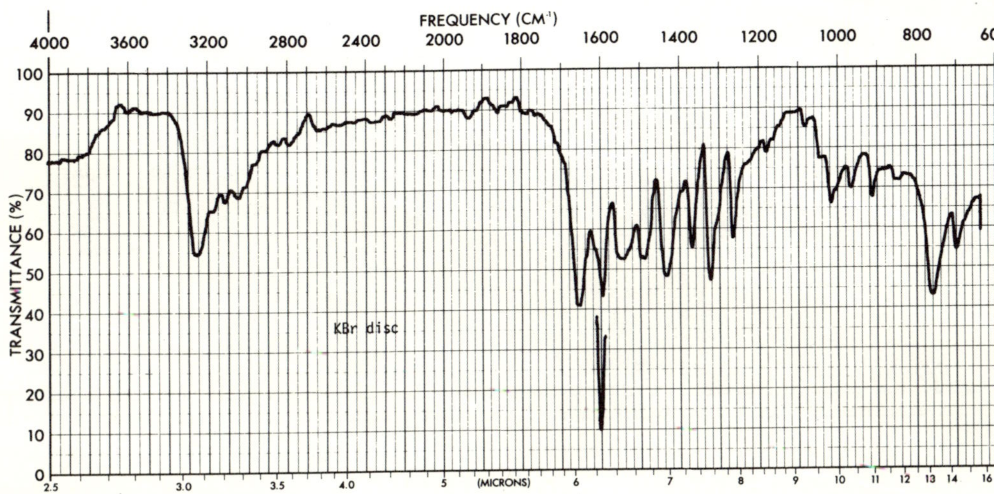

Compound No. 3

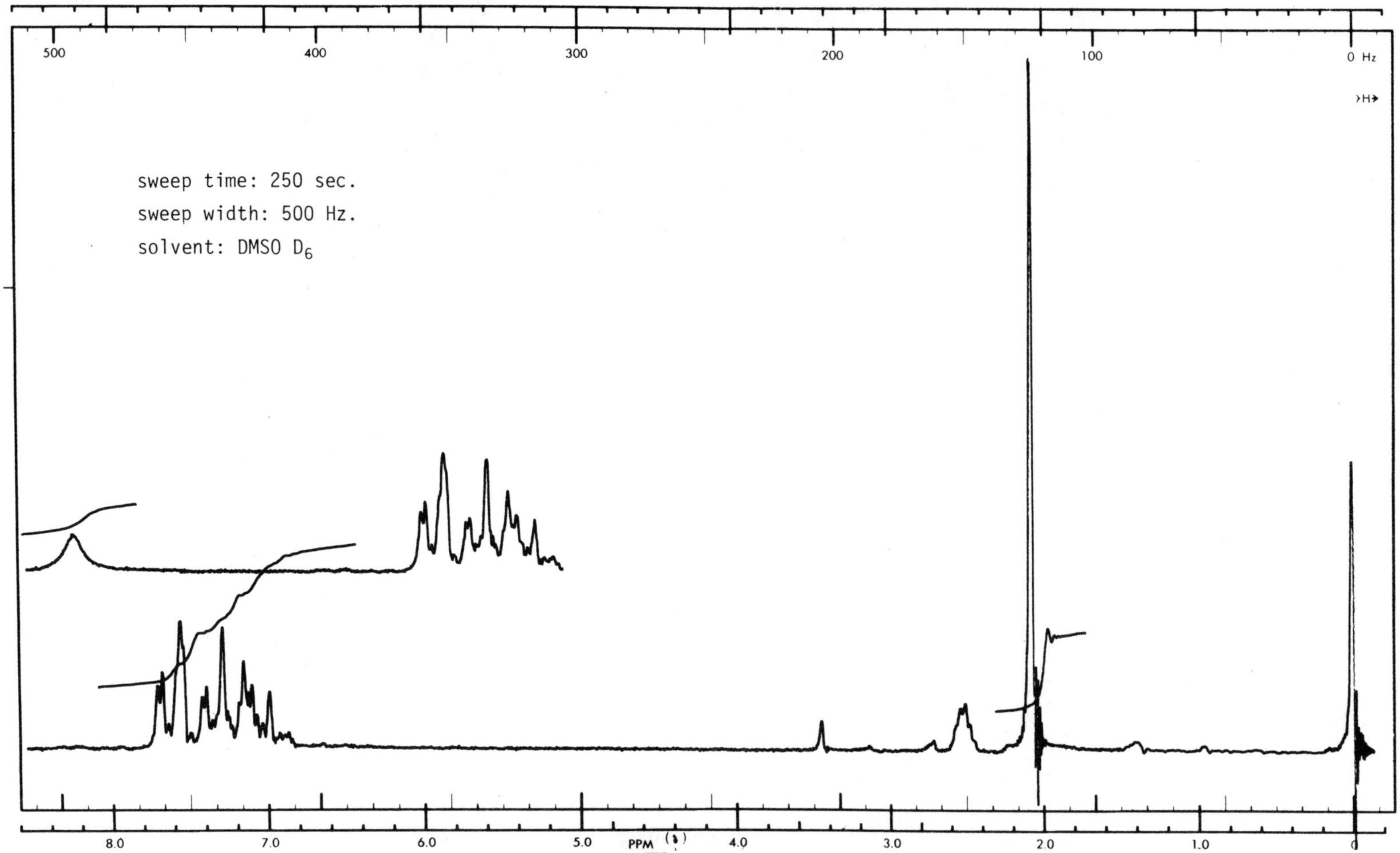

Compound No. 4

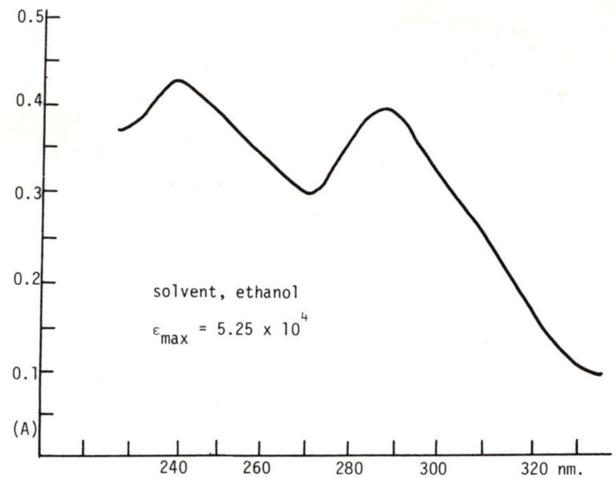

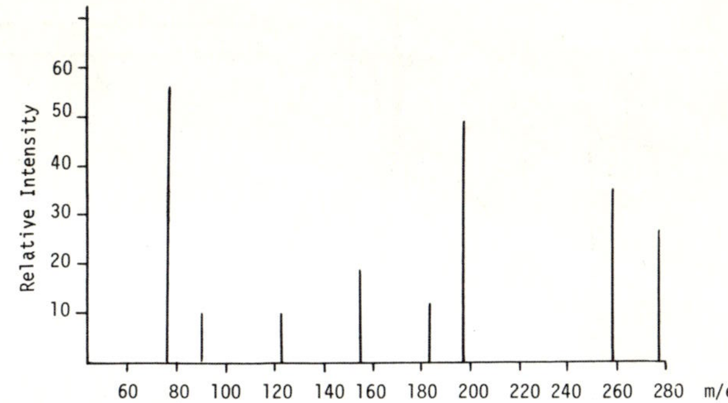

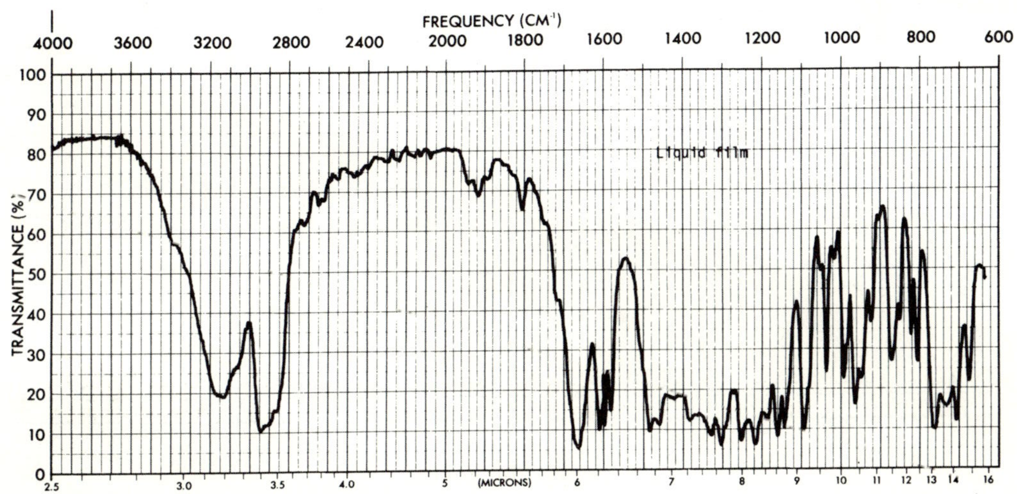

Compound No. 4

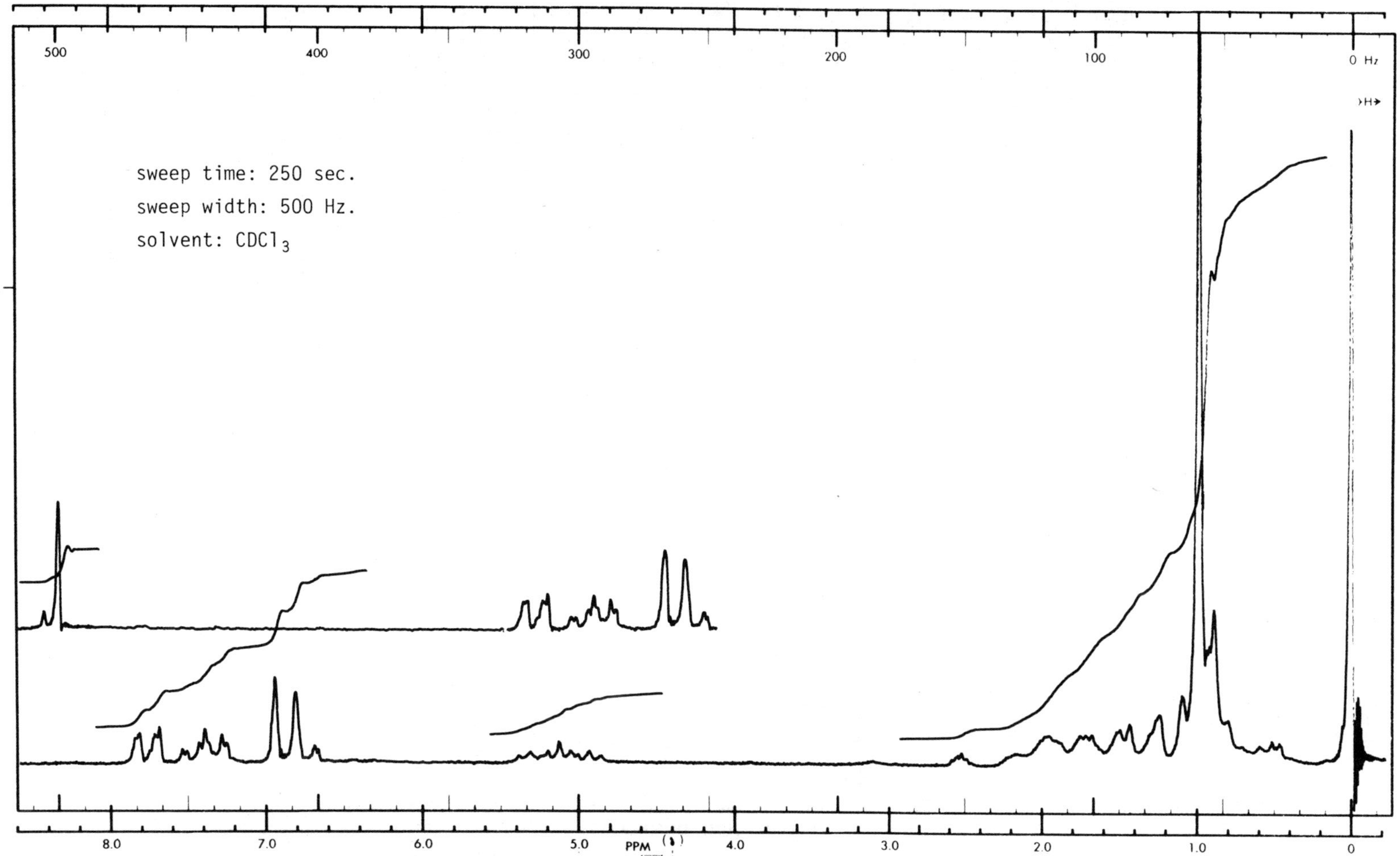

Compound No. 5

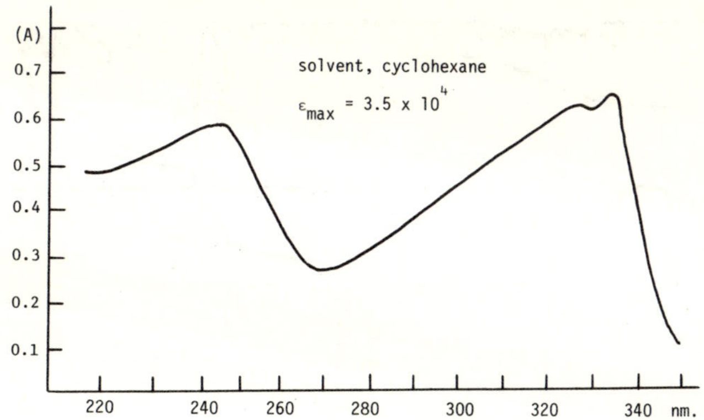

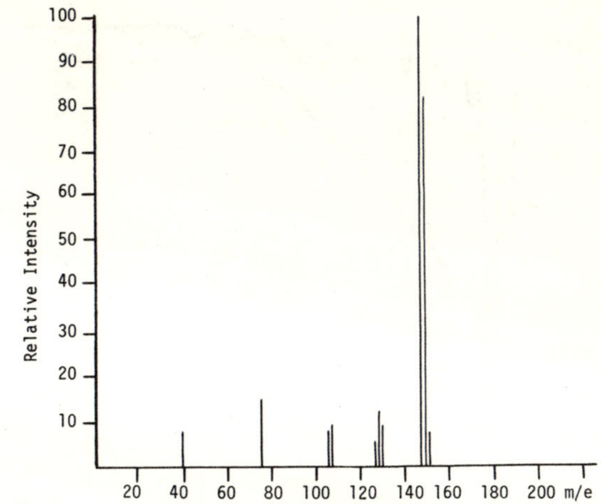

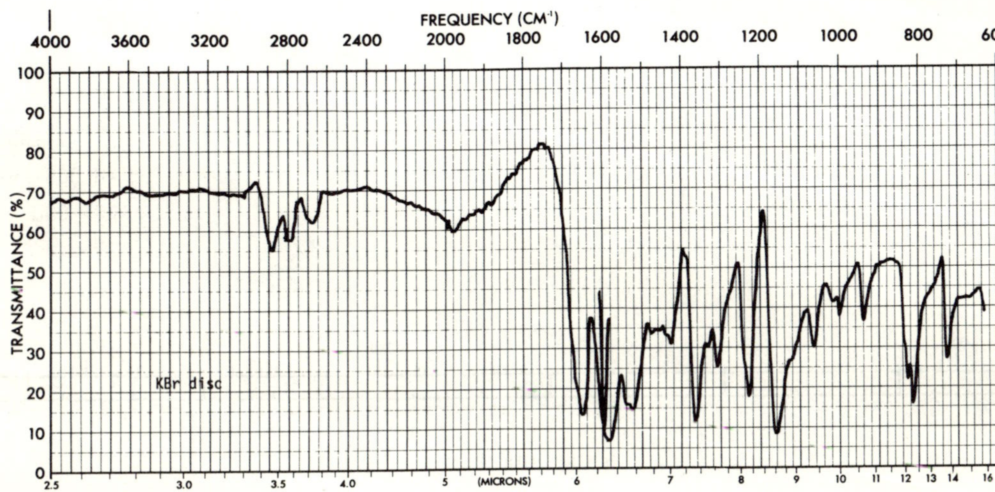

Compound No. 5

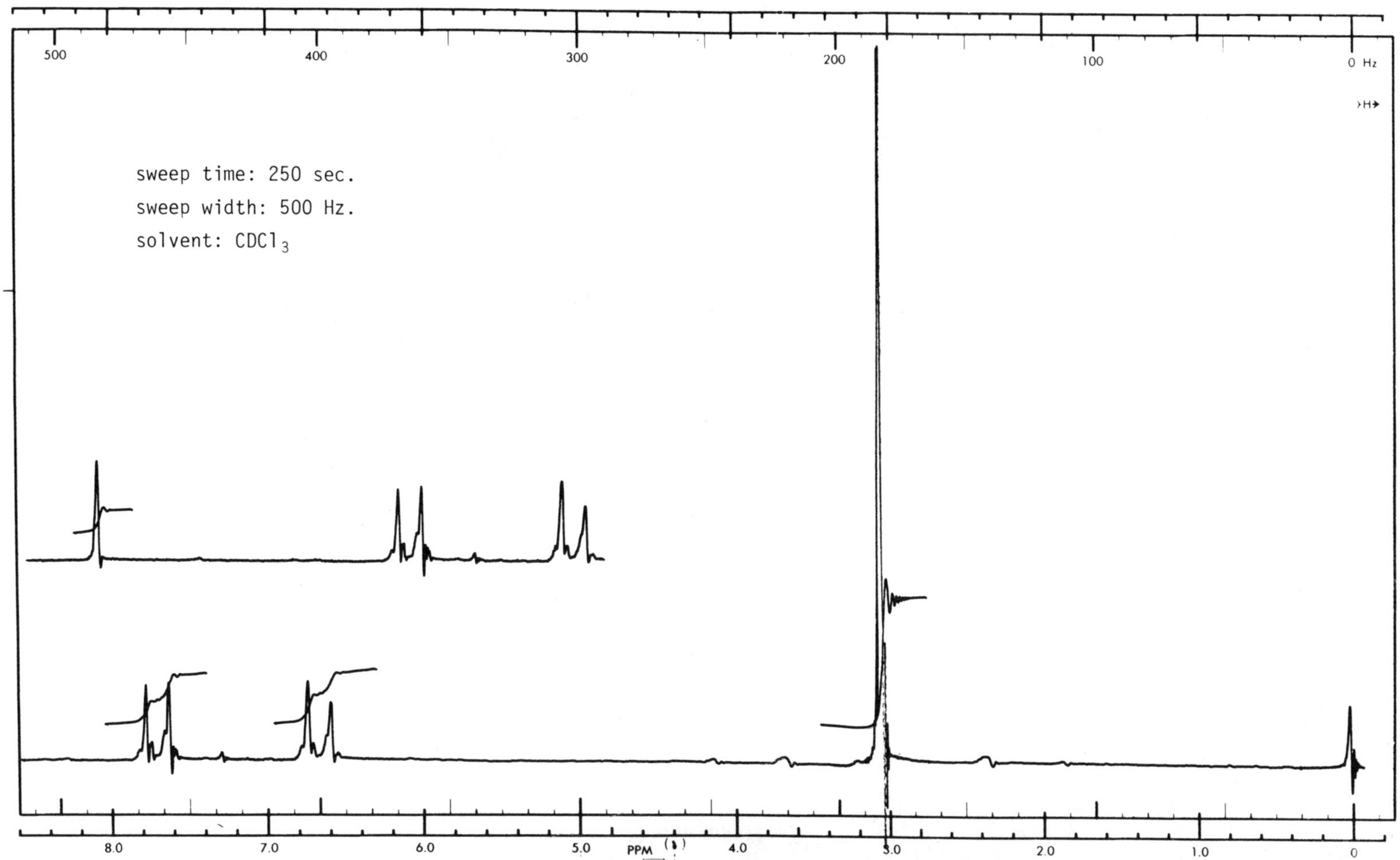

Compound No. 6

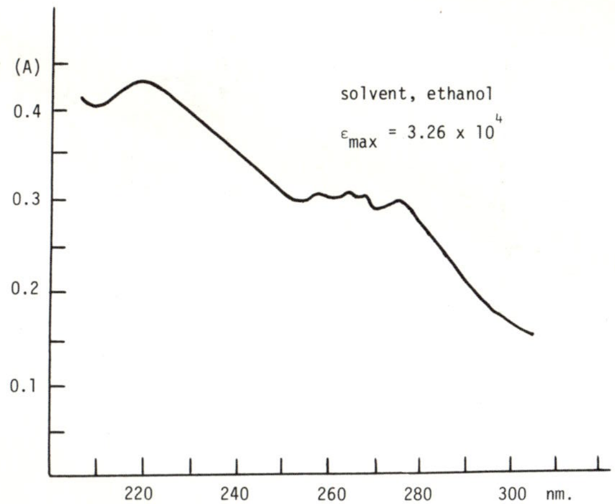

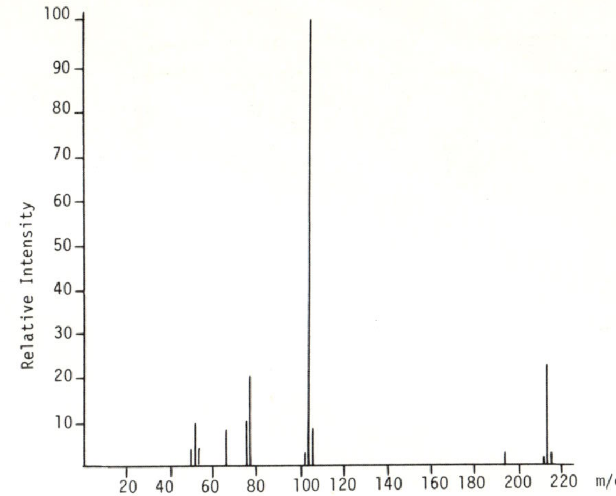

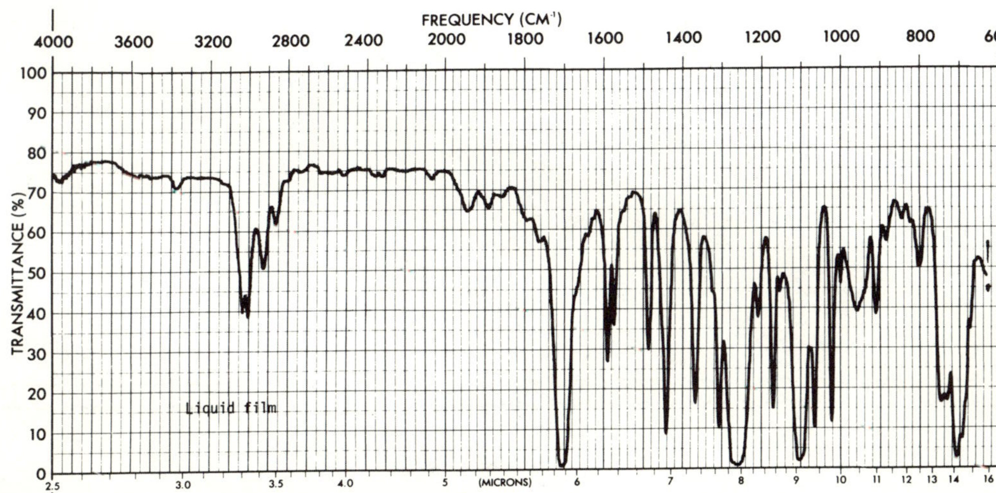

Compound No. 6

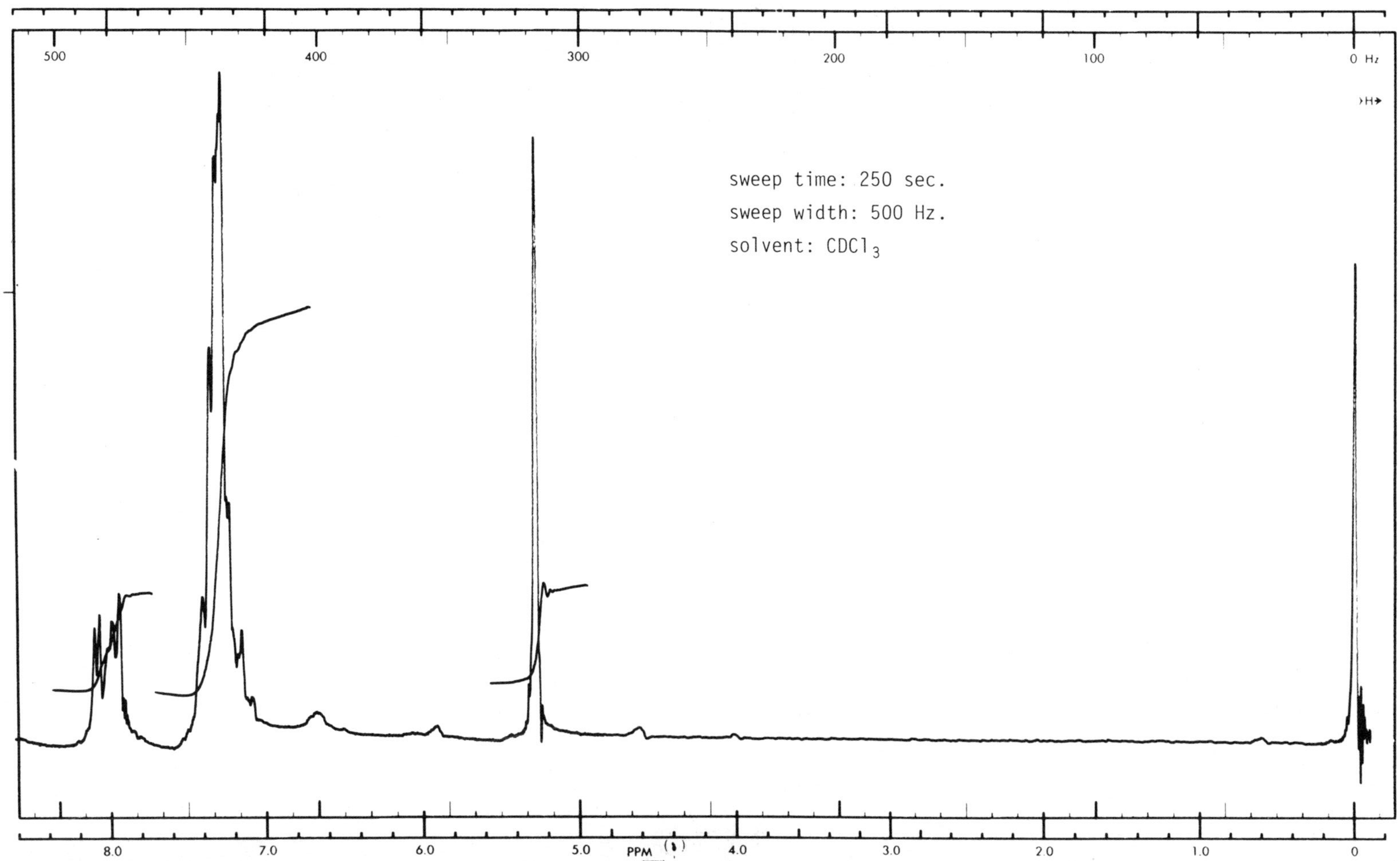

Compound No. 7

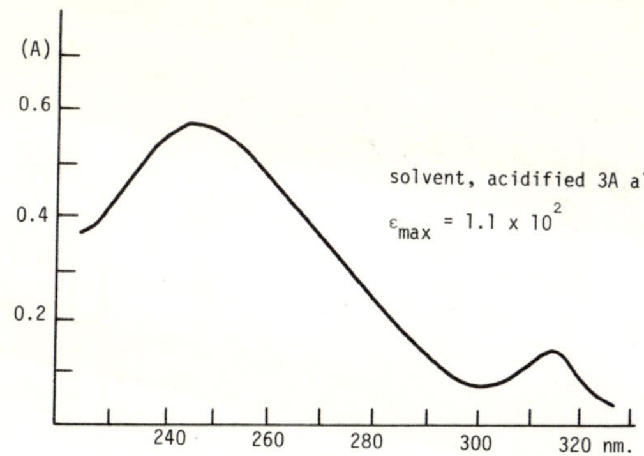

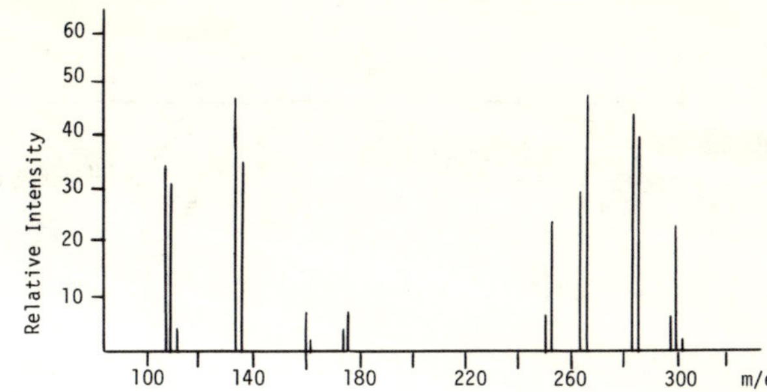

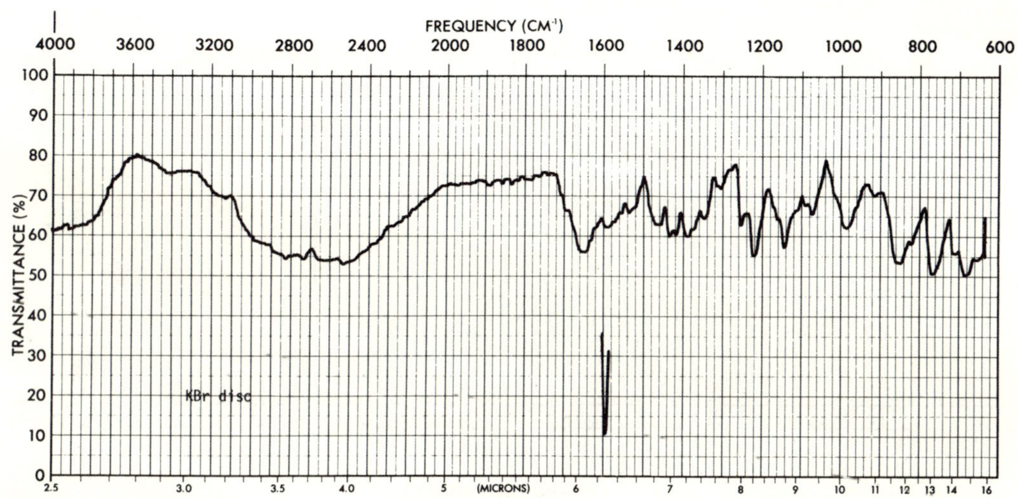

Compound No. 7

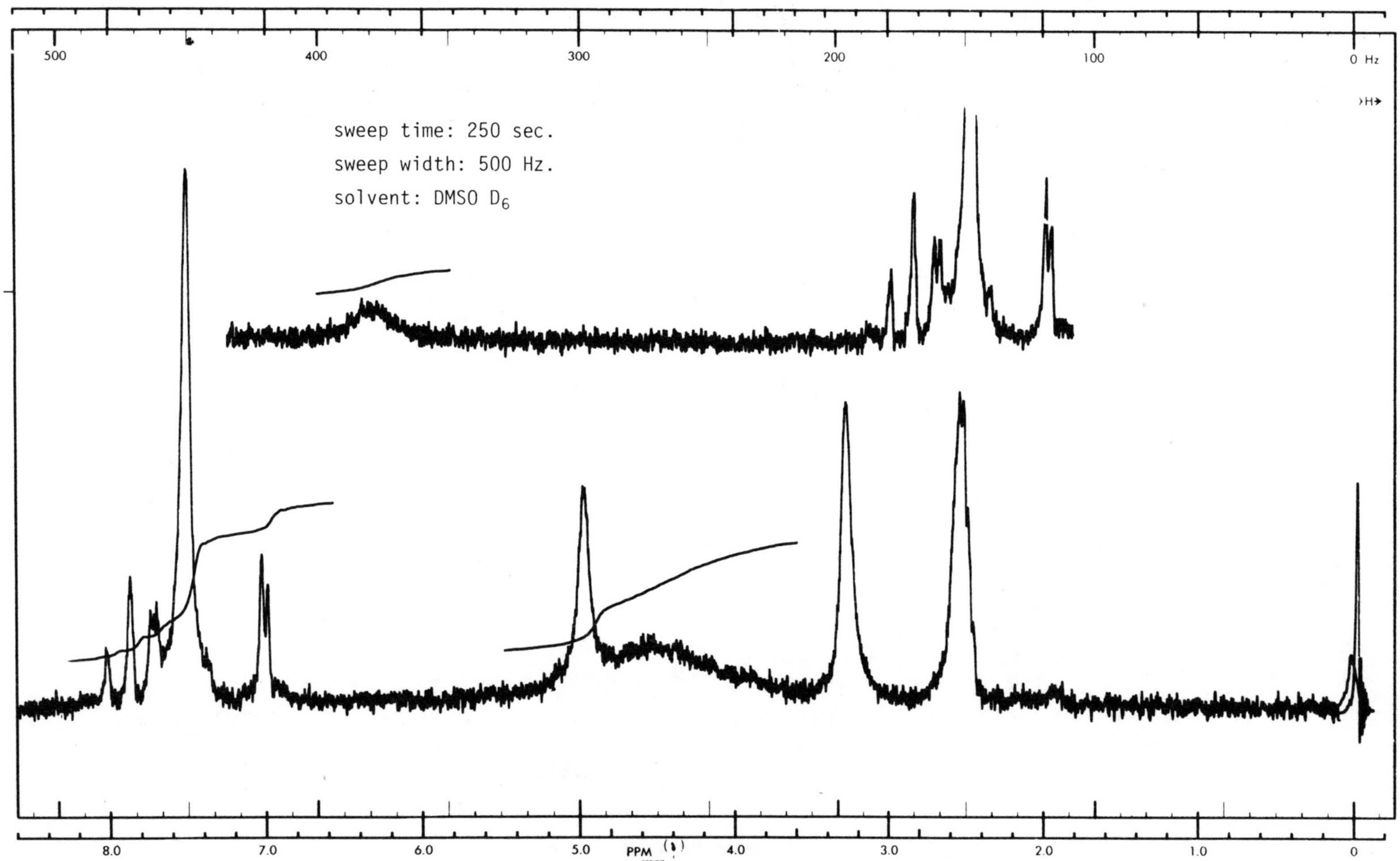

Compound No. 8

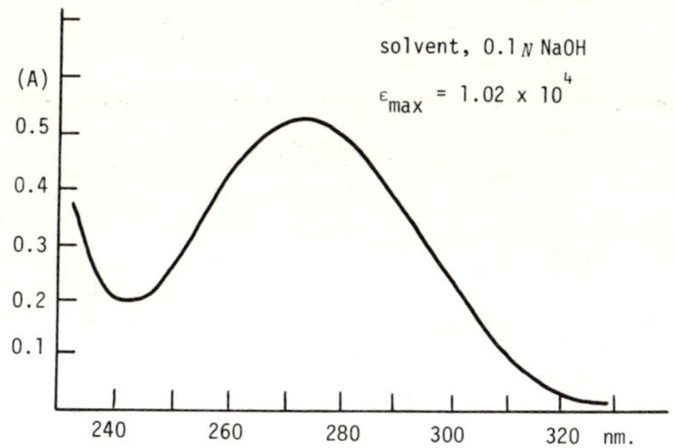

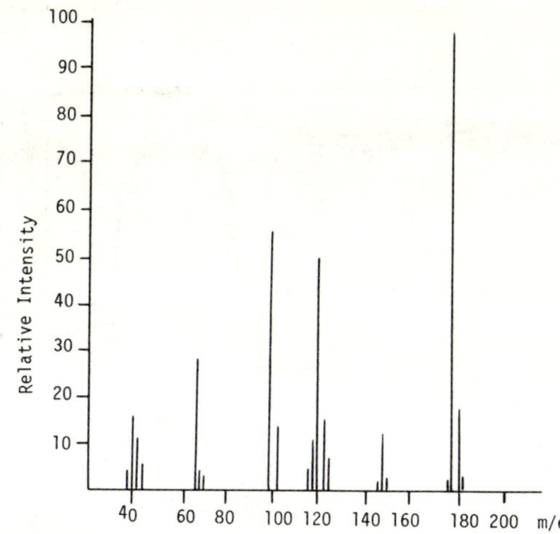

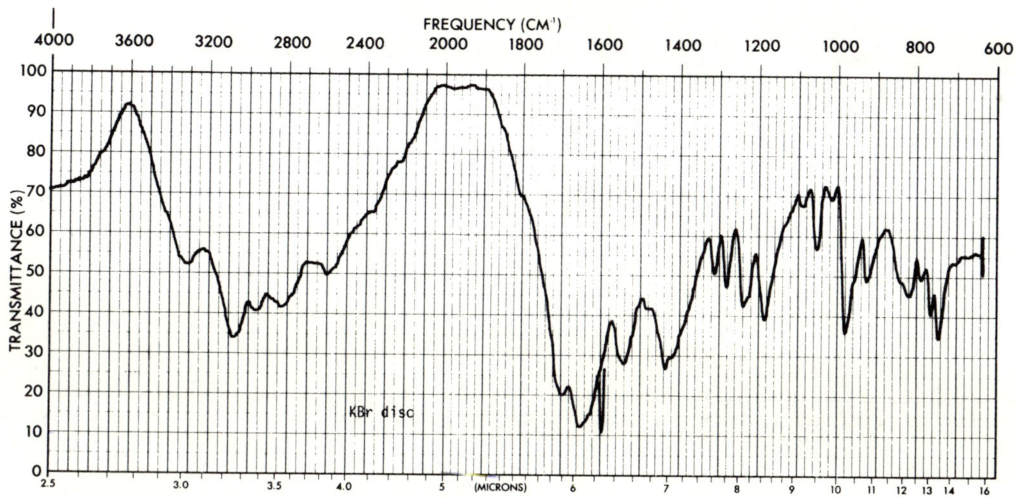

Compound No. 8

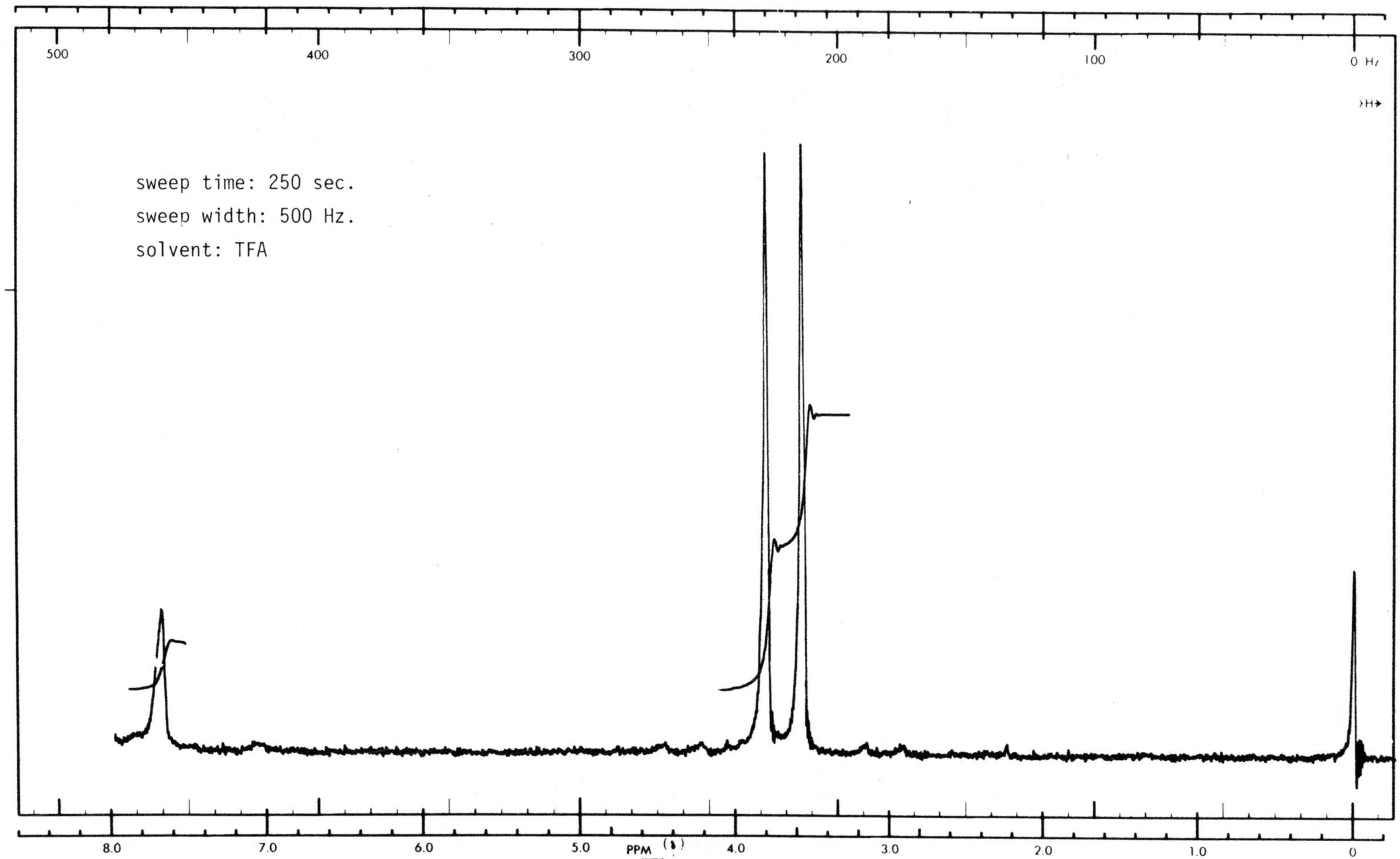

Compound No. 9

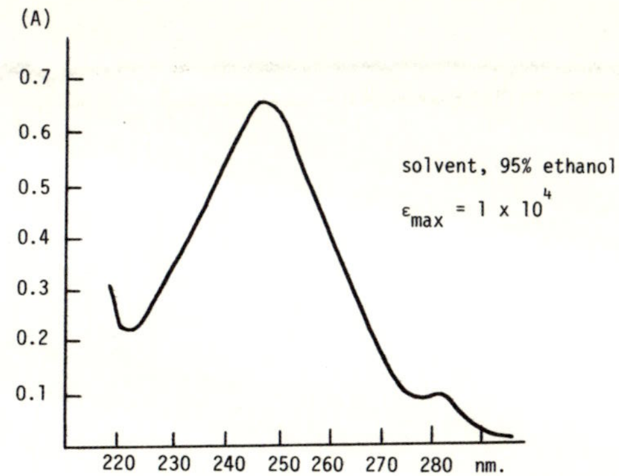

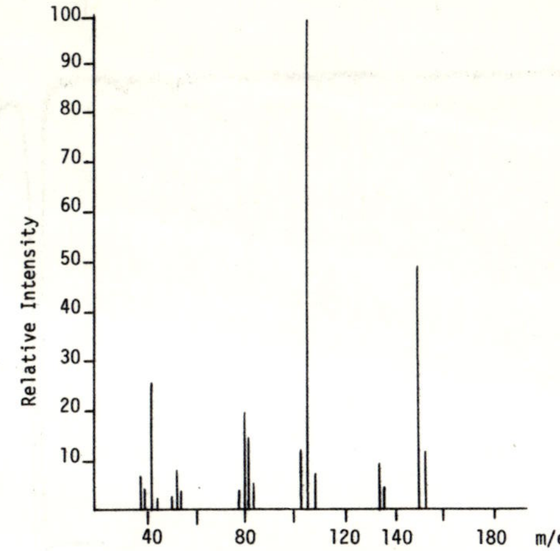

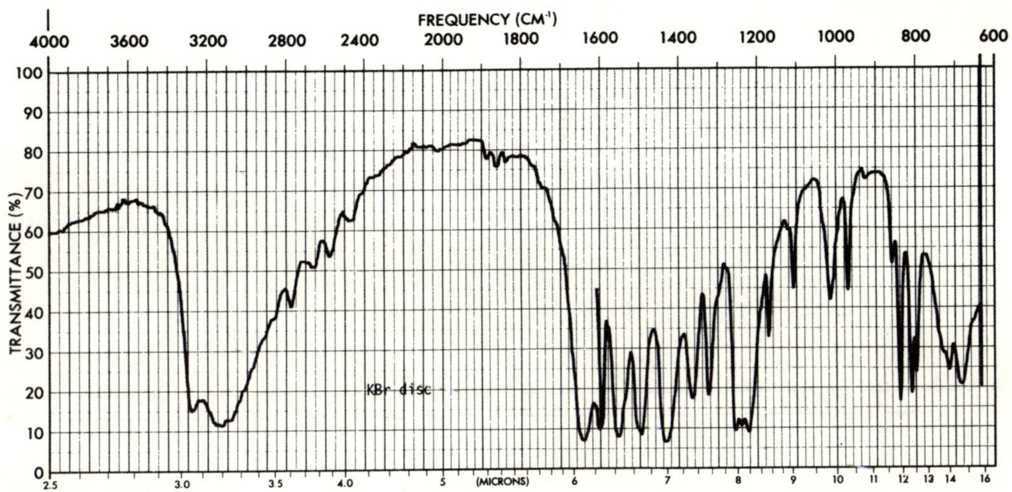

Compound No. 9

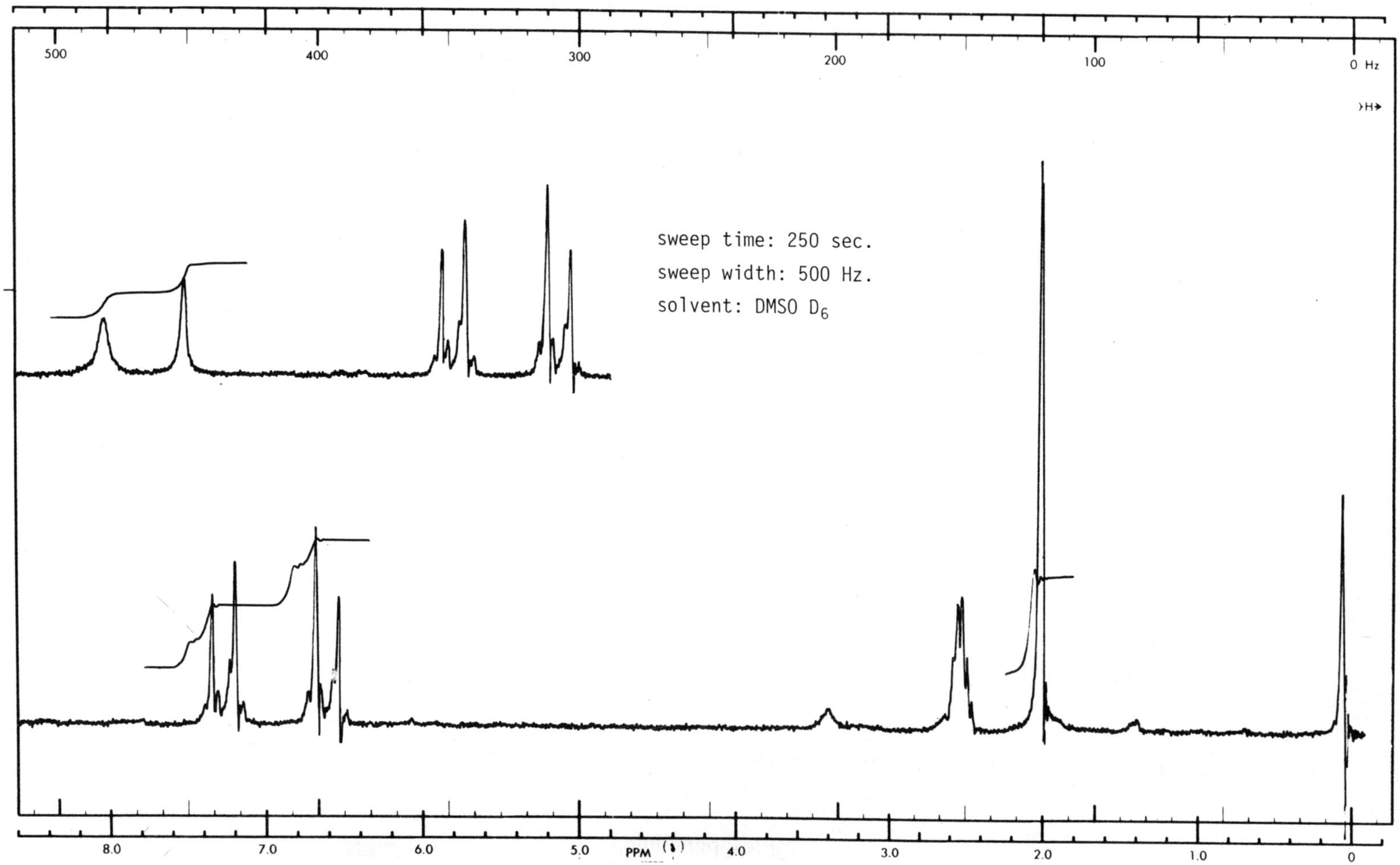

Compound No. 10

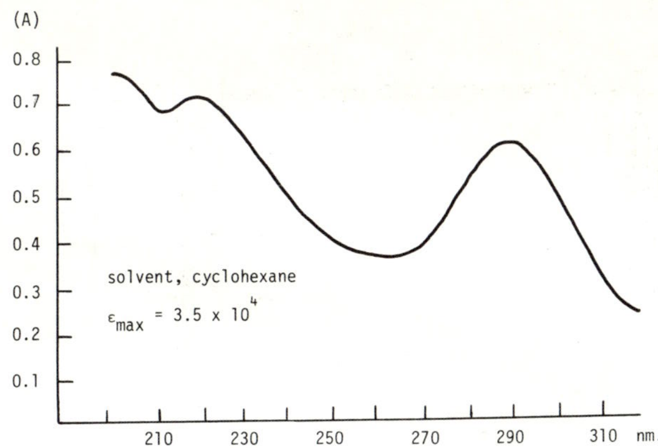

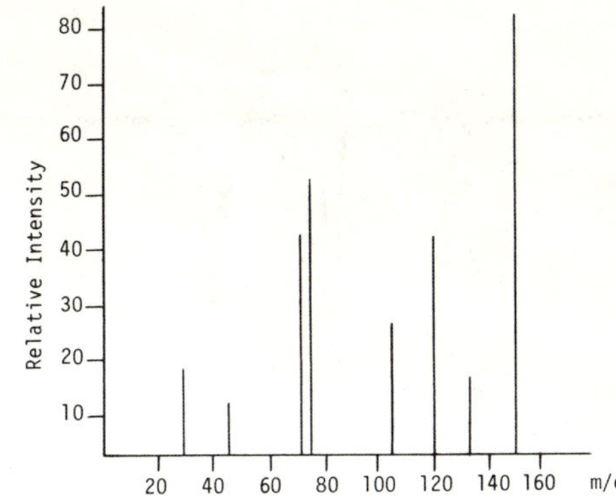

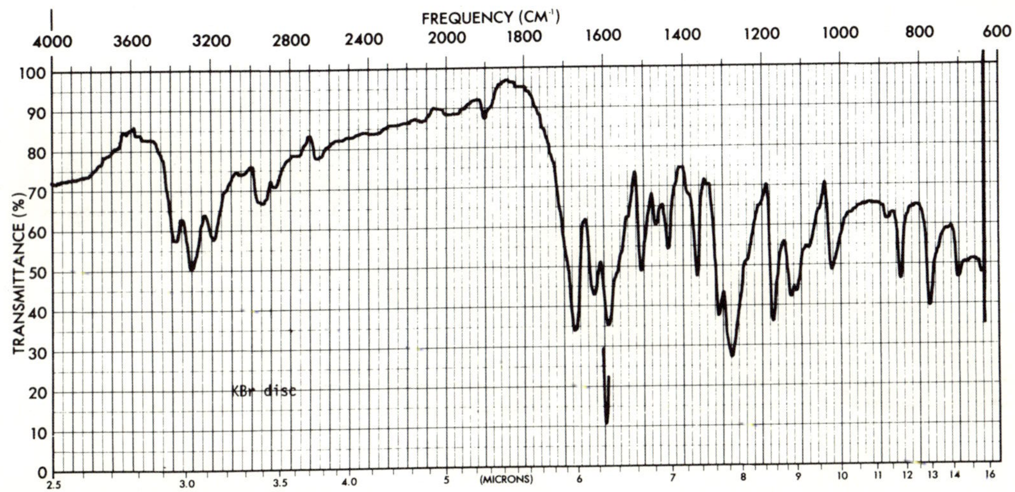

Compound No. 10

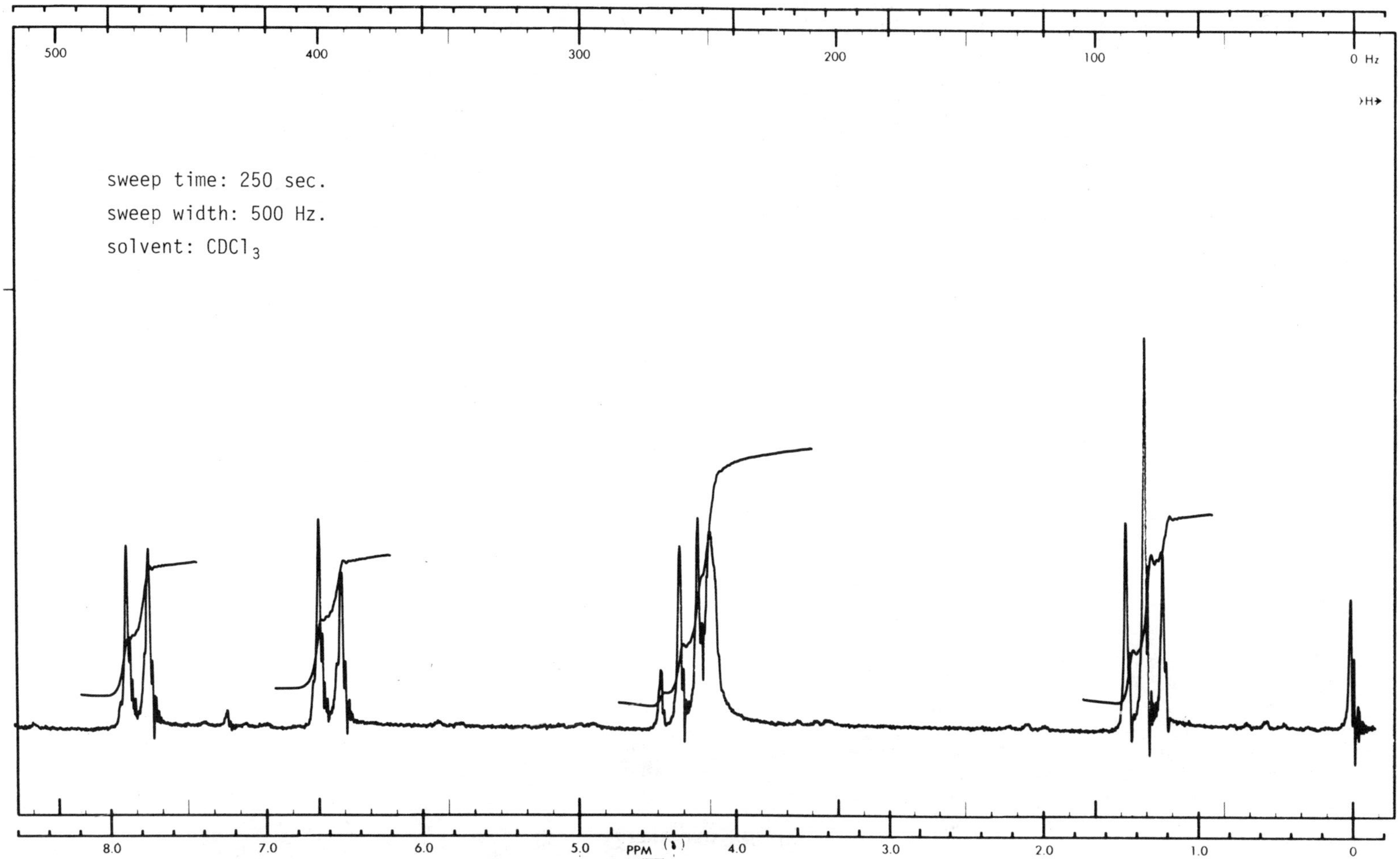

Compound No. 11

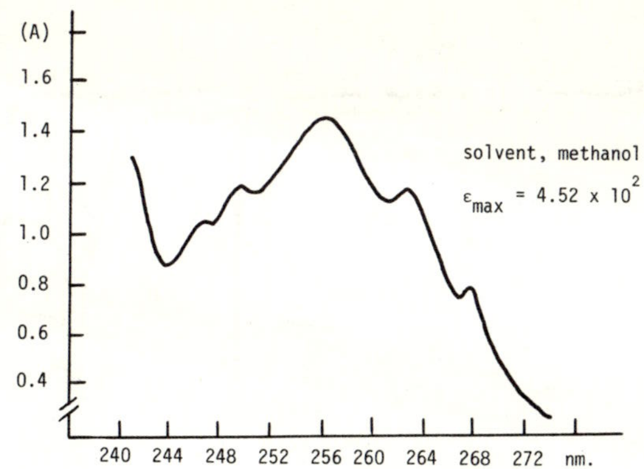

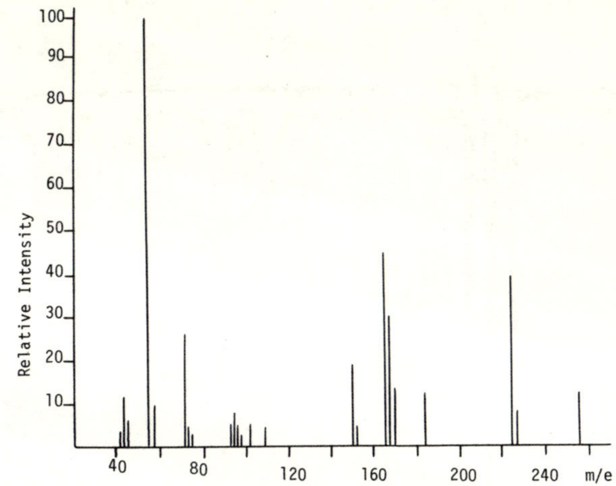

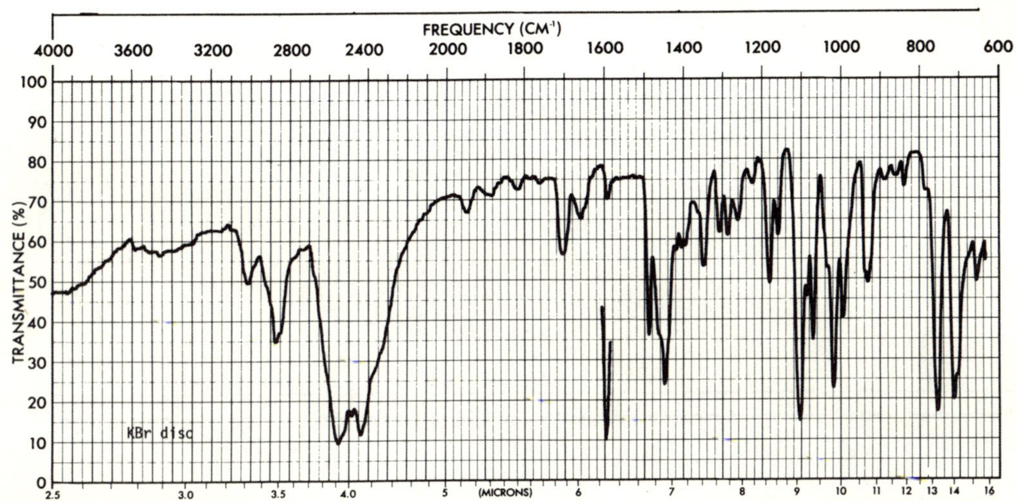

Compound No. 11

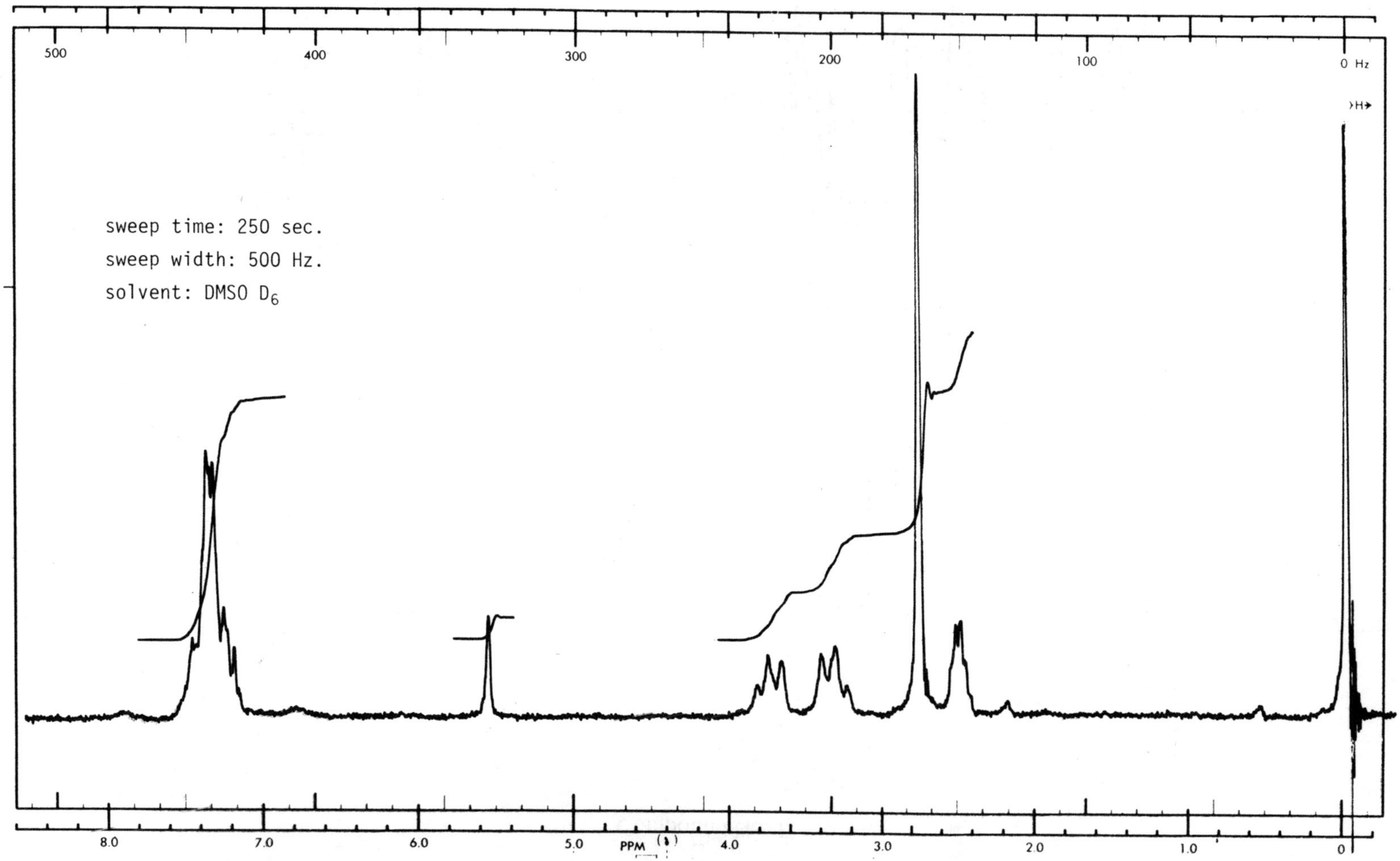

Compound No. 12

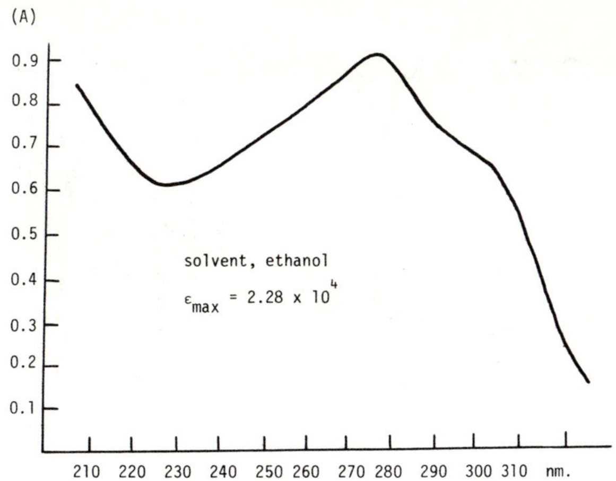

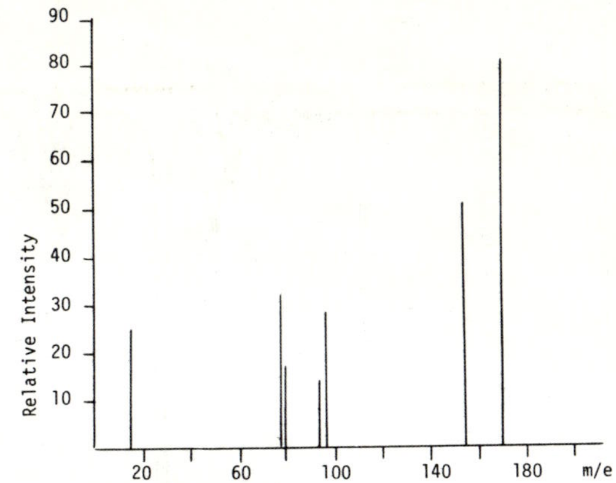

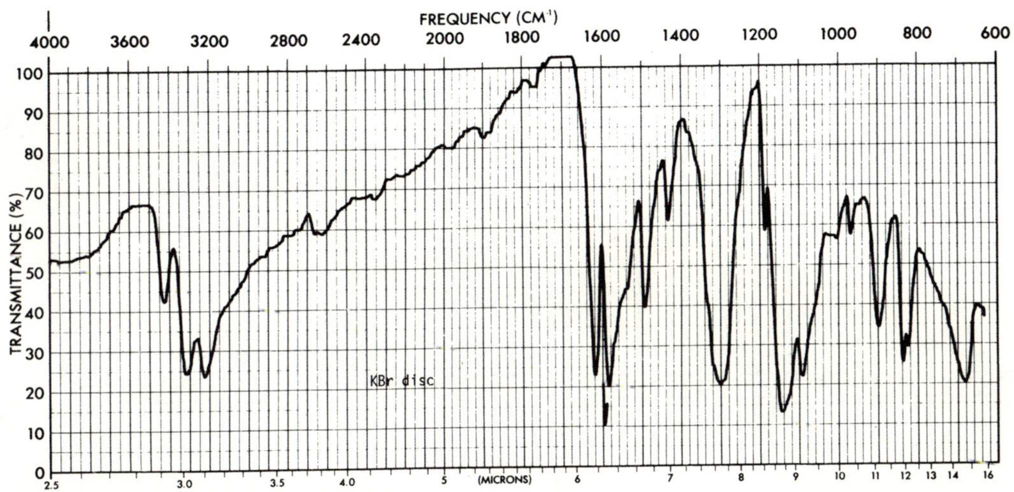

Compound No. 12

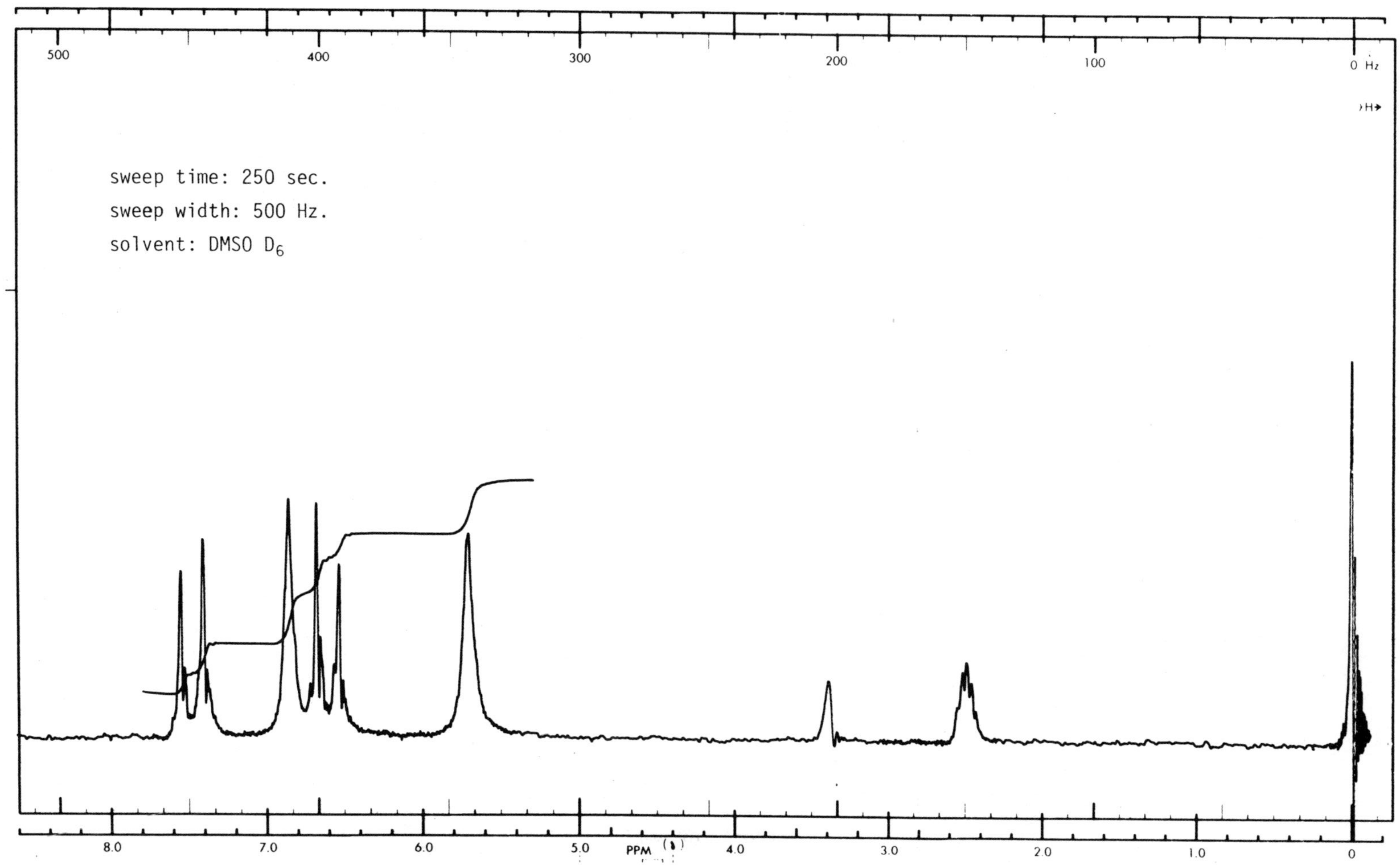

Index